The **Grea**

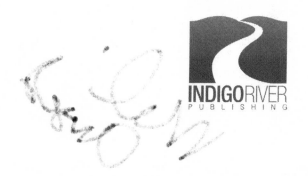

INDIGORIVER
PUBLISHING

The Grecian Garden

A Natural Path to Wellness

By Melanie Angelis MS

The Grecian Garden

Editors: Christian Pacheco, Earl Tillinghast
Cover Design: Joyce Walz
Interior Design: Lisa DeSpain
Indigo River Publishing
3 West Garden Street Ste. 352
Pensacola, FL 32502
www.indigoriverpublishing.com

Ordering Information:
Quantity sales: Special discounts are available on quantity purchases by corporations, associations, and others. For details, contact the publisher at the address above.
Orders by U.S. trade bookstores and wholesalers: Please contact the publisher at the address above.

Printed in the United States of America

Library of Congress Control Number: 2016932803
ISBN: 978-0-9972945-0-7
First Edition

With Indigo River Publishing, you can always expect great books, strong voices, and meaningful messages. Most importantly, you'll always find... words worth reading.

In this book, several terms will appear in bold type, indicating that they will appear in the glossary in the appendix. These will be great reference points for readers just starting out on their wellness journey and those who aren't familiar with medical and other wellness terminology.

Dedication

I dedicate this book to those with the courage to fight for
their dreams—those not afraid to challenge
the status quo and the diagnosis.

Acknowledgements

With utmost gratitude and respect I thank, Niko, without whom this book would have never seen the light of day. Thank you for editing and helping me capture the true essence of The Grecian Garden.

Thank you to my family who never gave up on me.

Thank you to my coworkers at Old Thyme Remedies, you are all a joy to work with.

Thank you to my clients, your stories have inspired me and I'm happy to be a part of your journey.

Thank you to Adam, Dan, Donna, Earl, Jason, and Christian at Indigo River Publishing for all your help in seeing the vision, tirelessly editing, and encouraging me along the way.

Thank you to the test readers, your attention to detail did not go unnoticed.

Writing this book was the most difficult venture I ever completed. The process of writing a book involves a lot of help from a lot of people and this book was no exception. I would also like to thank my Savior, Jesus Christ. I gave him the pen to write the story of my life a long time ago and he truly turned my ashes into beauty. I would not be a complete and whole person if it wasn't for His love and guidance overseeing my life.

Table of Contents

Foreword

Crushing pain wracked my chest. I could barely breathe. I paced my dorm room as thoughts ran through my head. *"Should I go to the doctor? This isn't really happening."* But it was, and as the tears rolled down my cheeks I noticed another symptom: left arm pain. What was happening to me? I was three months away from college graduation and I'd been ignoring strange symptoms for over six years, but this was different. I decided the pain was too unbearable not to at least get an X-ray. As I picked up my keys, my roommate walked in and asked me what was wrong. I started to tell her what was going on but she quickly interrupted me, telling me she would drive me to the hospital.

We waited there for four hours. I'm sure the nurses thought I was crazy. What 21-year-old has heart attack symptoms? They finally took me back and the elderly ER doctor asked me if I fell and hurt my shoulder. I hadn't. It was just a typical weekend out with friends Saturday night and teaching Sunday school that morning. After my short explanation, he sent me home with a diagnosis of bursitis of the shoulder and a prescription painkiller.

When the two of us got back to our dorm room, I made a turkey sandwich, took my prescription and a sleeping pill, and tried to get some rest. I woke up at midnight with even stronger chest pains and began freaking out. We returned to the ER only this time they took me more seriously, and I knew my journey was far from over.

CHAPTER ONE

Hungry for Answers

My **wellness** journey started way before I ended up in the hospital twice in 24 hours. Growing up, food was more than just breakfast, lunch, and dinner. Food connected me with my family roots and the sound of chopping, blending, and mixing was music to my soul. I loved nothing more than to drag a chair in front of the stove and cook with my grandma. If I stood on that chair I towered over the pots and pans and felt so tall being able to look my five-foot-tall grandma in her eye.

"That Melanie eats like she's got a holler leg," my grandmother would say. And it's true! I never turned down good food, and in our house that meant creamy mashed potatoes, home-style meatloaf, Grandma's coleslaw, corn bread, and spanakopita. I was completely immersed in two entirely different cultures in our household; we had my mom's Southern roots and my dad's Greek heritage shaping our every move—including the food choices we made. I not only learned the secret to making my grandmother's famous McCormick mashed potatoes, but also discovered how to make the most succulent lamb you'd ever taste. Food and I had a close relationship. By seventh grade, I was making dinner for our family of six every night. Some meals were just okay, but our family favorites were the Greek-inspired ones.

As my long-term relationship with food and family blossomed, I became very curious about nutrition. I especially liked to think of nutrition as prevention, and I realized that if I ate a certain way, I could prevent future diseases. This passion started a lifelong habit of reading about all things health-related. In high school, I gravitated towards the most nutrition-conscious information available to me like my mom's *Women's Circle*, *Women's Day*, and *Cooking Light* magazines. Their catchy slogans about weight loss, cancer prevention, and healthy cooking tips seemed truthful and easy enough. Make your sandwiches with whole wheat bread, add low-fat dairy products to your diet and ditch sugar for Splenda, things like that. I faithfully made all the changes necessary for a healthy diet by eating oatmeal with cottage cheese for breakfast and munching on baby carrots.

Despite all the reading, I left one important piece out of my picture of health: me. I was so out of tune with my own body that I didn't realize it was speaking to me through symptoms every day.

Stomachaches, overwhelming fatigue, and a funny coating on my tongue plagued me for a year before I started connecting the dots. Trying to keep my frustrations under control, I tried to make sense of my situation by justifying each symptom with the most logical of reasoning. Is antacid deficiency a real condition? Or maybe the answer to my fatigue could be found at Starbucks? What nutrient could I possibly be missing with my well-rounded standard American diet, sprinkled with feta cheese and doused in gravy?

I wanted a quick fix for my odd health problems, so I regularly checked the medicine aisle for ways to hide my symptoms. Sadly, doctors prescribed the same method—temporary reduction of the symptoms without addressing the underlying issues. It was round after round of powerful antibiotics and a diagnosis of the stomach flu each and every time.

I continued to read nutrition facts and apply them to my diet immediately, such as eating soy cheese with rye crackers and baking with spelt instead of wheat. The advice from my gastrointestinal doctor was simple: eat more fiber. On my way home I bought those little fiber tablets—another fail... No matter what wacky supplements I tried or how many bricks of soy cheese I ate, I kept expecting to see a complete turnaround in my health. Unfortunately, this was only the beginning of a long quest to find complete and true healing for my worsening conditions.

I thought the answer was out there but realized healing was only in reach if I could figure out what was wrong. After my bout of chest pain, I was diagnosed with a heart condition, which was possibly permanent, and painkillers were simply a Band-Aid. My joints ached and I couldn't concentrate on anything even if I did manage to sleep enough. I felt hungry all the time, yet nothing satisfied me. I had to take a break after anything as strenuous as making dinner, and I really felt like I had a terminal disease.

I desperately wanted answers, and after all the research, studying, going to different doctors, and trying medications and supplements, I had to come face to face with a part of me that realized, "I'm still not getting better. In fact I'm getting worse by the day." I felt so discouraged that I slumped down on my bedroom floor, feeling as though I had hit rock bottom with nowhere to turn. Curled in the fetal position with sharp pains wracking my body, it was in that moment I turned to the place I received strength from my whole life.

"God," I prayed with tears streaming down my face, "I need your help! I know you can heal me. Please help me get better."

I should point out that I grew up in a pew at church, and if we weren't running a high fever we were there every Sunday with dresses on and hair curled. My parents instilled in us a faith as sturdy as my Greek grandfather's seafaring legs. Whenever we were going through a tough time as a family, my mom would pull out the Bible and read its promises over us. She taught us to rely on God when our faith was strong so that we would already be used to talking to Him when our strength was weak, as it was that night on my bedroom floor. I got off the floor with renewed conviction that I would find out what was wrong with me.

Part of my challenge was discerning if nutrition information I read was true or not. I tried so many therapies, supplements, and foods to no avail that I decided to see a naturopath, a doctor who specializes in holistic care and preventative practices. She tested my blood, spit, and poop (not as awkward as you might think) and actually asked me what I ate on a daily basis.

No one had asked me that before.

After writing down everything ingested for a week, I realized how many burgers and cookies I ate. She also told me to follow the anti-**Candida** diet and gave me a laundry list of supplements. I tried limiting my sugar and starch intake as the diet required several times without success, usually thanks to Greek pastries at family weddings.

Finally the day came. I drove to my natural doctor's office to learn all of my test results. I remember holding that piece of paper, hoping I'd discover what was actually doing so much damage to my body. By this time I had been sick for over four years and I was really getting tired of being a medical mystery. I needed answers.

My problem had a name: **Blastocystis hominis**—a protozoan that had overstayed his welcome, living in my gut the whole time. What? You mean to tell me after five years of going to doctors and being told I either had food poisoning or the flu and none of them found this out before? Thoughts started racing through my head: "If I was treated for a parasitic infection could I have actually felt normal during college?" And what about my heart? Would I have gone through tortuous chest pains if the parasite had been found sooner?

My thoughts were interrupted by the naturopath asking if I had traveled outside of the country. Years prior, I traveled to Ecuador on a mission trip—in that moment feelings of bitterness and resentment overwhelmed me. I realized there wouldn't be a quick fix for my health, regardless of what specialist I saw. It just wasn't fair! I shared Jesus with Ecuadorian villagers, and they inadvertently shared parasites with me. After a few moments, I managed to look at the positive side. At least I now had some direction. I knew what was wrong with me and, armed with my bottles of herbal powders and potions, there was a ray of hope that began to quickly dim.

I kept trying to follow the anti-Candida diet and similar protocols for months without improvement. As for the supplements, all the alternative health practitioners I visited each had new regimens and herbs to try, all of them hoping for a magic bullet (or at least a gullible patient). I wondered if they were doing any good at all. My digestion was shot, so how did they expect me to handle 16 capsules of just one of my supplements each day, plus six other herbal formulas to take several times a day? Exhaustion followed me wherever I went and I felt drained physically, financially, emotionally, and spiritually.

I found myself curled up in pain yet again, crying and pleading with God to heal me or lead me to more information that could help me. In the midst of all of my pleas, He whispered in my ear, "This isn't just for you." It was at that moment that I realized all that I had gone through and all that I was going to go through had nothing to do with me, but with the countless other individuals who need a transformation in their health. My shuddering sobs faded, taking the stabbing pains with them. I felt a quiet peace come over me and knew God heard my prayer. He would guide me on my journey to wellness, placing the resources and people I needed in my path. While I was sure I could eventually find answers, I wouldn't keep them to myself. This experience served as training for everyone I met with baffling conditions or desperate health situations.

I continued to study nutrition and health books around the clock, but I also began researching symptoms and diseases I never had. Instead of just looking for my own personal answers, I began learning how to help others. I wanted to know for sure which therapies, supplements, and foods were restorative and healing.

My questions were answered a week later in front of my mom's bookshelf. As usual, I was quickly scanning the shelves for new cookbooks or recipe magazines when I saw *The Maker's Diet* by Jordin Rubin. The book chronicles Jordin's recovery from life-threatening illness to vibrant health. Everything in my being resonated with his story and perspectives on nutrition, and applying Jordin's principles became an important first step for me.

I devoured *The Maker's Diet* in one sitting and soon noticed a subtle difference in my health. I was hungry for more truth and found what I was looking for when my sister Eleni learned about Dr. Weston A. Price, one of the sources Jordin often quotes. In reading his sentinel work *Nutrition and Physical Degeneration*, I learned that our health affects our descendants for generations. Here at my fingertips was information that could not only change my own health but that of my family and even the world!

I was able to fine tune what works in **alternative medicine** and apply it to myself. After eliminating the parasite and healing my gut, my chronic fatigue was a thing of the past and I began to feel like a new person. After my last echocardiogram, the cardiologist congratulated me because I no longer had a heart condition. This newfound energy and passion led me to leave my teaching career to study health and nutrition full time. As I began my first graduate classes in **holistic nutrition**, it became so much easier to understand research articles and decipher the value of various conventional and alternative therapies. Alternative medicine is often looked down upon, but the field advocates prevention and healing in a way that is much healthier for our bodies than limping along with our symptoms masked by powerful pharmaceuticals. Yes, there are completely worthless supplements and treatments out there that only work because of a **placebo effect**—just the hope of getting well is enough for some people. The solution is to treat each person individually with a tailored natural medicine protocol addressing their core issues. Getting healthy requires a holistic, whole body approach, which is why simply taking random supplements doesn't resolve a health concern. Looking at the big picture is key. The purpose of this book is not to treat, cure, prevent, or diagnose your current health situation but to introduce solutions and sustainable lifestyle changes. Gently shifting a few habits will accelerate your journey to wellness. The same lifestyle changes that turned my life around are at your fingertips.

After years of cooking, changing my lifestyle habits, studying advanced nutrition, and working with clients, my answer really came from a place I didn't expect. It didn't come from the blend of science and holistic techniques I learned in my postgraduate training—it came from looking deep inside myself and listening to what my body needed. Ultimately, it's not the science or **meta-analysis** of **double-blind research studies** that will make us healthy. Knowing all the nutrition science in the world isn't going to make anyone get better. It's the action that counts. In my younger days I applied the latest media-hyped health headlines to my diet and it got me nowhere. The answer to our health isn't in magazines, dieting, or low-fat cottage cheese. It is our connection with ourselves, which is sometimes the last place we look to give love. The answer is not out there floating in space. It starts at the core, the center of our being. It starts at finding a personal sense of purpose for wanting a better path for ourselves. Why you should make the change for a healthier future is a question you will need to answer before embarking on any health program, because without that motivation your plans will fail. Maybe it's for the love of your children and the desire to age gracefully so you can be active grandparents, or maybe you'll decide to walk a more holistic path for the benefit of your future children. Maybe you are struggling with health challenges and you know it's time to fight back. Until we are willing to take these first initial steps to define our goals, none of the instructions in this book will make a difference.

> Ultimately, it's not the science or **meta-analysis** of **double-blind research studies** that will make us healthy. Knowing all the nutrition science in the world isn't going to make anyone get better. It's the action that counts.

After dramatically healing my body through the natural techniques I will share in this book, a passion ignited in me to help other people. A friend found the healthy tips and recipes I'd started sharing on my blog, and asked me to teach at a women's conference shortly thereafter. I brought along business cards with my new company name and logo: "The Grecian Garden." It was the manifestation of the answer to my prayer and allowed me to share a message of hope with anyone with a health challenge. I continued to teach classes and also began consulting. As each person filed in my office door with mysterious ailments, I would pinpoint root problems and get them started on a complete turnaround in their health.

As I work on it, that little whisper from years ago seems loud and clear as to why this book needs to be written. I don't want another 21-year-old to be diagnosed with a heart condition or a young child to needlessly suffer with food allergies. Living a preventive lifestyle affects you, your family, and eventually your community as you share what you've learned (and will learn). I'm going to challenge you to do things for your health that are not about losing weight, but about avoiding the roller coaster of health trials that I went through. You may have already been on that roller coaster, or maybe you are in the midst of your symptoms as you read this. Make sure you're strapped in, because we're going to acknowledge the superficial—weight and appearance—but blow past that to the core of why we're sick and what we can do about it.

Health fads have come and gone in the four years since I started writing this book, but certain truths remain. What have my clients achieved by applying my principles to their lives and what can you expect? Changes like increased energy and alertness, weight loss, less pain and inflammation, clearer skin, freedom from digestive disorders, disease prevention, fewer doctor visits, and more.

If you are feeling a little overwhelmed, let's use a real life example to help you better understand. Imagine we are doing a makeover on your house. We already know it can only be done one step at a time and that an organized approach will give us the best results. We may need to get rid of old unwanted items, sanitize cracks and corners, and maybe even knock down a wall or two. But first we need a game plan. What do we want the house to look like when we are done? We need to decide the best place to begin. We could start in one room or one corner of a room and continue like that throughout the whole house until everything is the way we want it. Some of you may only have a few cobwebs to brush away. Others need a hazmat suit to dispose of hoarded habits. The end result should be our focus and reward. Changing your health is the same process. What is your goal and what actions are you taking today to get you there?

Let's play out this imaginary scene a little further. We are going to go step by step and layer the foundations of a healthy diet and natural health techniques for a totally transformed you. Taking any one of the topics presented in this book can improve health dramatically and result in a positive transformation. This isn't just about food, although formulating and consuming a healthy diet is an important step. There may be something you don't know about affecting your health. Sometimes the negative emotions we harbor can be just as toxic as junk food or wrongly prescribed pharmaceuticals. Being conscious of what we are doing to our bodies on a daily basis is one of the most important concepts I can teach you.

So, what exactly is our first step on this very practical journey? We need to know how and why we're sick. Genetics, environment, and other underlying causes are major factors, but the simplest answer is right under your nose—your mouth. It's time to make those almost 2,000 meals per year count by choosing to heal with every meal. We'll even discuss the right way to exercise, go hunting for clean water, and learn the best herbal and **homeopathic** remedies. There may be a massage or **reflexology** appointment soon on your calendar. I realize you're not going to eat broccoli with every meal until I convince you that there is no alternative to choosing a healthy lifestyle. Just kidding about the broccoli.

> It's time to make those almost 2,000 meals per year count by choosing to heal with every meal.

Action Steps: Do your goals and actions match up?

Before moving forward, take a closer look at your health and motivations.

- Write down your current state of health. Have you had to modify your activities or alter your lifestyle because of your health?

- List any ongoing symptoms you may have. Rashes, colds, or frequent headaches. Do you catch everything that's going around?

- What is motivating you to be healthier? Your children? Your current symptoms? Write it down and be specific.

CHAPTER TWO

Distorted Perceptions

"We came to see Melanie for our son who seemed to be having some behavior issues. She found a sensitivity to corn and gave him some food enzymes. When we removed corn from his diet there was a night and day difference. We noticed improvement in his behavior right away and we are still amazed!"

—Amanda Hayes

We are going to dive into many areas in the upcoming chapters on how and why to implement certain lifestyle changes for optimal health. But, before I tell you about the true causes that can wreak havoc on your health we need to take a look at truth or the lack thereof within the nutrition community. We've relied on false studies and outdated diet mythology for too long and developed a distorted perception on perceptions about what healthy foods truly are. With countless diet types and all sorts of health information available to us, why are obesity and heart disease still increasing? It's time to find out how we got here so we don't make the same mistakes going forward.

What Went Wrong?

When I read that Americans aren't getting enough vegetables in their daily diets [1], that we don't exercise enough [2], and that high stress lifestyles are the norm, I correlate it with the following facts: 50% of

Americans have been diagnosed with some form of arthritis [3], one in 88 children are somewhere on the autism spectrum, over 27 million Americans have heart disease [4], and 600,000 people die from cancer every year [5]. I don't know about you but those numbers freak me out! They don't freak me out in that I'm paralyzed with fear; rather, those are the numbers that keep me moving, keep me drinking bone broth, and keep me learning more about my body. I don't want to be just another statistic, nor do I want you to be.

Media Mix-Up

Statistics and trendy one-line explanations of complex research can be misleading, and we can be inclined to make rash decisions based on messages from familiar and usually reputable sources. As activist Daniel Vitalis says, "There's a reason TV is called programming."

The classic example is in fast food commercials where people seem energized and healthy after ingesting nutrient-devoid, artificially fortified foods. Another example we've become accustomed to seeing is drug advertisements where patients are asking their doctors for drugs based upon specific symptoms or diseases. They make it look normal to ask for specific prescriptions and take them for the rest of your life. Let's not even mention all the side effects they list, but simply note how programmed we become when it comes to going to the doctor. A doctor's appointment isn't always about pills. It should be about finding the root cause and not just covering up symptoms with band-aids (drugs). Some appointments with my clients aren't about putting them on a new supplement but rather reinforcing lifestyle or dietary changes so they continue to see improvement.

Miracle Cure

Before we learn about distorted nutrition perceptions, we need to examine our own viewpoints and beliefs about health. I know that mine is skewed towards natural medicine to such an extent that I don't even have a bottle of Tylenol or any other drug in my house.

I'm not saying it's wrong to use prescription drugs, have surgery, or try **acupuncture**, but *every point* on the continuum could be compromised by quackery. Get suspicious when it just seems too good to be true. Depending on the situation, I find myself between lab work and alternative medicine, taking what's best from both sides.

> ### Where are you on this continuum from traditional to alternative medicine?
>
> Rx Drugs –
>   Surgery –
>   Invasive Testing –
>   Lab work –
>   Healthy Lifestyle –
>   Herbs and Supplements –
>   Natural/Alternative Medicine –
>   "Snake Oil"

Starting at the far left of the continuum, unnecessary surgery or prescriptions won't improve anyone's health. Let's take bone loss for example. There are many drugs on the market promoted as viable solutions for bone loss, but the side effects of creating a biological patchwork quilt with calcium, magnesium, and bisphosphonates are intolerable for some. As one study states, "Osteoporosis is a preventable disease, not an inevitable consequence of aging." [6] So much for receiving a new titanium skeleton once we hit menopause. Bones are a living matrix of minerals, including trace amounts of boron and selenium. Healthy fats such as cod liver oil guide minerals into order in the bone matrix. Strength

> The journey to natural health involves commitment, lifestyle changes, creating new habits, and modifying what you put in your mouth.

training maintains the matrix's shape, but taking one prescription drug will not reverse someone's osteoporosis. [6, 7]

Veering to the far right end of the continuum is snake oil. I'm sure you've heard about a miracle packet of powder that dissolves in water to shed weight, improve the complexion, heal your neighbor's kid of autism, and cure your aunt's fibromyalgia. Sounds too good to be true, right? There are thousands of "priceless" products like that because we want to believe our miracle can happen without effort. The journey to natural health involves commitment, lifestyle changes, creating new habits, and modifying what you put in your mouth.

Probably the hardest out of all of the above is changing food choices. I'll dwell on that in detail, but please know I don't recommend any quick fix health products. I'm reminded of a client who tried everything to lose weight. When she came to me she was frustrated and had lost all hope. After testing her we found food sensitivities, Candida, and adrenal fatigue as stumbling blocks to her previous attempts. I couldn't believe it when she sent me before and after pictures. She changed her diet, healed her adrenals, and subdued her infection. She lost 70 pounds, beamed with energy, and looked years younger.

Our Distorted Perceptions

A cereal box says you can eat chocolate sugar balls and get all your daily calcium needs. We haven't truly made the connection between food and medicine.

Everywhere we look, advertisers hope to pluck our consumer dollar out of our hand and into their pocket. Typically, if a food needs advertising it isn't really food. I often like to ask myself while reading or watching an ad, "Who's paying for this anyway?" Not someone who is interested in our health, that's for sure! We don't have to be a nutrition expert to know there is a warped view about what truly healthy food is. Take a look at the grocery carts of those around you at the checkout and you will find plenty of low fat, diet, or "lite" foods with ingredients lists longer than the articles in People magazine. A cereal box says you can eat chocolate sugar balls and get all your daily calcium needs. We haven't truly made the connection between food and medicine. We're pretending that our sugary fortified cereal is good healthy food when it's identical to taking an unfortified cereal with a cheap multivitamin. We've all seen the ad where they make high fructose corn syrup by simply squeezing those little corn kernels hard enough until a golden delicious sweet sap pops out. *Advertising distorts reality.*

The cornerstone for living a healthy life is to eat real food. But what is real food? I used to buy into the media and advertising lies as a sold out junk food-aholic, but I once heard Paul Nison say, "It's not what you put in your diet that counts, it's what you leave out." This was one reason why my body took so long to heal. I never stuck to an appropriate healing diet long enough and always found ways to sneak junk food. I also failed in the food department by not listening or paying attention to my own body—who better to ask what was going wrong, right? My body did not send vague signals. I would feel an overpowering urge to eat sugar and would be riding an emotional rollercoaster all day after splurging. It wasn't nicotine or meth, just Candida and parasites craving the empty calories that fed them. What your body feels after eating something is more relevant than any article written about that particular food, herb, or supplement. So many supposedly energizing foods made me want to curl up and take a nap.

> "It's not what you put in your diet that counts, it's what you leave out."

Inconvenience

We think it's inconvenient to make or eat real food. Rachael Ray has been teaching about 30-minute meals for years and showing us how to make three-course meals each night of the week, yet we wait 40 minutes to be seated at Olive Garden. In our society, we have an abundance of food that we easily take for granted. We begin to believe that it does nothing for us other than stop our stomachs from growling. Years of just keeping our tummies full and misleading dietary advice has made us numb, unconscious, and literally disconnected with our diet. We're eating fake food and it's making us codependent. It's much the same thing in many relationships, the other person makes you feel good temporarily, even though you know that they are bad for you long term. In all relationships, we want to be heard and nurtured with our best interests kept in mind, and dietary habits are no different.

When heavily processed or "fast" foods first came on the scene, people were not eating them daily from the moment they abandoned the milk bottle for a French fry. They might have had one TV dinner a week or splurged on fast food once a month. Although fast food is never healthy, at least this method gave the body time to recover from the empty calorie, nutrient devoid mistake. How come, as science and technology has increased, so has sickness and disease? I blame the media, advertising, and false nutrition studies, and we'll look at some of those studies in the next section, but stay encouraged.

One step in making healthy choices for a positive effect on our health is to commit to a few small changes. As we'll see in the exercise chapter, instead of adding a cheap supplement or purchasing the latest flavored vitamin water, try walking 15 minutes a day to increase life expectancy while decreasing life time medical costs.[2] What's another small change that will result in glowing skin, increased energy, and improved digestion? You knew fruits and veggies were going to come up sooner or later didn't you? One study found that 60% of Americans aren't getting the daily recommended amount of fresh produce. [1] Walking and making a glass of vegetable juice are just two simple steps to reiterate how truly convenient it is to take care of our bodies.

There is no quick fix, pill, or technique to rescue us from the standard American diet, but the change to a more helpful diet is possible if we take one step at a time. Commit to a change and make it a habit before moving on to the next level. We can't simply pretend the standard American diet never existed, but over time our new habits will become effortless. Before you know it you'll be enjoying a grass-fed steak, eating avocados and olives for a snack, and finding a local farmer to get eggs.

Diet Mythology

To make matters even more disheartening when it comes to nutrition is the abundance of misinformation that is available. Poorly done scientific studies create dietary myths. When it comes to statistics and research, little details matter. The culprit is sometimes the messenger (media). Translations of results are dumbed down to a catchy phrase, and most sound bites can be taken way out of context. What stands out the most are the headlines. "Fruit will make you fat" will be stuck in our memories better than, "Refined foods with high fructose corn syrup contribute to weight gain." We don't get a Get Out of Jail Free card so easily either. We often try to find weight loss strategies based on our own theories and fantasies. As long as it vibes with our own thinking we believe it no matter what the claims.

> The best advice is to avoid foods with health claims on the label, or better yet avoid foods with labels in the first place.
> –Mark Hyman

Many scientists believe that chronic disease only came about once we ate high-fat diets at the turn of the twentieth century, along with fewer grains. Unfortunately for those scientists, the data gathered by USDA was at best a guess until World War II. The more reliable statistics for the next 25 years documented soaring diagnoses of heart disease and plummeting amounts of animal fat consumption. Dr. Ancel Keys noted the increased fat contents in the American diet during this time, but the simple explanation is that our "heart-healthy" vegetable fat consumption doubled from 1949 to 1976. [8] In the 1950's, Keys led the world to believe that heart disease existed because of cholesterol and a high-fat diet. The problem with Keys' research was that he selectively chose seven countries out of the twenty that he analyzed (cherry picked) and didn't account for confounding variables—differences among studied people that could make study data less accurate. [9] Dr. Keys paved the way for margarine and canola oil to hit industrialized nations supermarkets and what was the result? A nation suffering from heart disease.

Cholesterol: Friend or Foe?

Cholesterol was an easy target, but even famous heart surgeons like Michael DeBakey failed to find a link between cholesterol levels and heart disease in their patients. High cholesterol levels are linked to all sorts of disorders nowhere near the heart, and those patients don't die of atherosclerosis more often than anyone else does, even when given high-cholesterol diets. [10] Contrary to popular belief, high-cholesterol diets don't increase blood cholesterol levels significantly, as even Keys pointed out in 1952. The research simply didn't show that increased fat increases cholesterol or even that increased cholesterol leads to atherosclerosis or heart disease. The American Heart Association wrote a report admitting this in 1957, but by 1960, the organization published a two-page paper without references but in support of a low-fat diet. [8]

In the late 1970s, half of researchers were still skeptical that enough evidence existed to link saturated fat with heart disease. That's because they were correctly looking at the problem from a preventative health standpoint—teaching healthy people how to tweak their diets to stay healthy—as opposed to an acute approach of hurriedly saving them from surreptitious heart disease. This meant that data disproving dietary fat hypotheses from isolated monks, Irish immigrants in Boston, Swiss farmers, and more groups was rejected. Keys responded that the peculiarities of those primitive nomads had no relevance to diet-cholesterol-coronary heart disease relationships in other populations. Over the years, similar results were skewed, and random statistics from specific ethnicities were touted as cause and effect relationships. [8]

I say all this not to make you paranoid about anything a doctor or scientist tells you. Good research disproves wrong theories. For example, after a large and well-constructed study on post-menopausal estrogens in 2002, the scientific community realized that the heart benefits of (non-bioidentical) hormone replacement therapy didn't exist after all and that such "preventative" care was increasing cancer, heart disease, stroke, and dementia risks! [11]

In the 1990s, increases in fat consumption in Japan, Spain, and Italy mirrored what researchers already knew about the French—diets high in fat don't lead to a population with higher risks for heart disease. More specific studies, such as the Framingham Heart Study, Stamler's MRFIT study, and Taylor's Harvard study all showed that people on low-fat diets were no more likely to live longer than anyone else. Dr. Castelli noticed that mortality levels increased as cholesterol levels decreased.

Although I'm sure my exposé on cholesterol and fat is fascinating, please take them with a grain of salt—literally—because the last myth to discuss is the low sodium myth. I'm certainly not telling you to go eat fast food because all that fat, salt, and cholesterol is good for you. The source of your food matters so much that I'm devoting the next chapter to it. What should you do if told you have high cholesterol? Know first

> "In Framingham, Massachusetts, the more saturated fat one ate, the more cholesterol one ate, the more calories one ate, the lower people's serum cholesterol...we found that the people who ate the most cholesterol, ate the most saturated fat, ate the most calories weighed the least and were the most physically active."
> —William Castelli, MD, Director, The Framingham Study

that cholesterol is like the firefighters of your body. They make it to the scene to help repair damage. What caused the damage and what we need to fight is **inflammation** which can be caused by infections, heavy metals, and other environmental toxins. Aim at the inflammation, not at the cholesterol.

Salt

As we left the hospital with my grandma after her low sodium level almost killed her, the nurse reminded Grandma to eat a 1,000-milligram sodium per day cardiac diet. Why was the hospital continuing to instruct her to lower her salt intake after I watched her not salt her food for 15 years? I knew that salt is important for specific biological functions, so you can be certain I stocked my grandparents pantry with both Celtic and Himalayan salt on the way home. How did the low-sodium diet begin, and is there any truth to it?

Let's start with what we know: sodium is essential for life. Unrefined, natural salt helps regulate blood pressure and the water in our bodies. It is an essential part of plasma and the extracellular fluid that it travels to transport nutrients between cells. It nourishes the glial cells in the brain that support memory-making neurons and is necessary for muscle function.

Before we go any further, it's important to note that most people are consuming way too much sodium from processed foods. Indisputably, this practice is harmful to your health. The type of salt used in convenience foods is mostly processed sodium chloride, not Himalayan or Celtic salt high in trace minerals. Let's dash the sodium myth.

What research caused us to replace our salt shaker with those artificial flakes with more colors than a crayon box? Volunteers ate a diet high in fruits and vegetables and low in salt and *sugar*. Guess what? Their blood pressure decreased! That's right, the low-sodium theory evolved from one lonely study hiding in the cupboard behind the salt shaker. Firstly, we shouldn't listen to any scientific study until two others confirm it. Secondly, we eat a lot more sugar than salt in this country, and low-sugar diets decrease blood pressure to healthy levels too. [12] Salt became the blood pressure villain while sugar toxicity was limited to discussions about weight loss.

One of the best research examples comes from the *Journal of Hypertension*. The study examined sodium excretion because the kidneys are the main organ interacting with salt to influence blood pressure. Sodium levels in the blood and urine were compared between two native Brazilian tribes and non-Indians. I know, I just love some native cultures, but I gravitate toward these studies because it's easy to say, "We'd all be healthier living in the jungle" without looking up the research. I believe it's harder to interpret studies from patients already in the Western healthcare system because of all the possible toxins and variables we can't control.

Anyway, high blood pressure, cholesterol, and high blood sugar levels were also compared between the three groups. Researchers hoped to show that the most primitive tribe had healthier results because of a low sodium diet. The study was successful in showing that cholesterol, obesity, blood sugar, and blood pressure were all lower in the more primitive tribe, but these results did not correlate with sodium levels. [13] The primitive tribe was healthier and it had nothing to do with salt. Subsequent studies show that low sodium diets can actually increase the risk of death from cardiovascular disease, but increased sodium doesn't increase the risk of high blood pressure, cardiovascular disease, or a quicker death. [14]

Obesity

"Is that fattening?" "I can't eat that or I'll get fat." We've been told for decades that sedentary lifestyles and overeating would cause weight gain. Americans eat less red meat, eggs, and fat now than in the 1960s. Our cholesterol levels have fallen, but unfortunately the evidence does not suggest that these decreases have improved our health. The percentage of Americans who smoke has also dropped dramatically, but this hasn't been enough to significantly reduce heart disease. Throughout the world the rate of diabetes and obesity has been increasing at an alarming rate. With the official recommendation to eat more carbohydrates and less fat, we've seen a third of the population struggle with weight gain. Directors of disease prevention at NIH expected obesity to decrease as individuals removed high-fat, high-calorie foods from their diets. Unfortunately that also is not the case as we are eating more, particularly carbs and "healthy" grains. [8] We have demonized saturated fat to bring more carbs into our life as a nutritional Savior. We also demonized fat, slandered complex carbs, and we are now trying to undermine animal protein with the vegan movement; truth is we've been blaming the wrong culprits the whole time: white sugar, white flour, and processed, unhealthy vegetable fats. Of course, that doesn't mean you should start every morning with a bowl of bacon strips and call it a gluten- and carb-free salad.

By the late 1970s, the argument that carbohydrates caused chronic diseases instead of fats had lost to the more politically expedient theory that it was only the lack of fiber that made refined grains unhealthy and inflammatory. Clinical trials have yet to prove that fiber magically transforms processed wheat any more than healthy dietary fat causes chronic disease. [8] Makes you wonder about all the advertising from cereal companies about how Americans need more fiber. It's necessary, but we've been told to eat more fiber to help our colon and heart to the point that there is wood fiber in our foods. I don't see any increase in health by eating like a beaver.

> We've been stuffed with grain like cattle being fattened for the slaughter and are still asking for more powdered sugar to be sprinkled on top.

I'm not trying to say that fixing the current health crisis is as easy as substituting a fat for every carb, but no one is at a healthier weight because of the studies processed food companies are paying to produce. Unlike the quacks of yesteryear promising the world with the next revolutionary product, these studies carry the weight of well-known food or health brands. They are harder to ignore. It doesn't take intimate knowledge of how carbohydrates affect insulin and glucose in the body to understand the causes of obesity. We've been stuffed with grain like cattle being fattened for the slaughter and are still asking for more powdered sugar to be sprinkled on top. If you follow the My Chart to get all the grains the USDA recommends, you would have a blood sugar spike six to 11 times a day. That would take a lot of coffee and five-hour energy drinks to overcome. It's no wonder we as a society need so many substances to stay awake or fall asleep.

Practically speaking, when you eat a piece of bread, whether white or whole grain, it's a simple sugar by the time it hits your small intestine. The pancreas releases insulin to transport the glucose from blood to cells. Sugar is toxic to blood vessels and organs, which is why it receives preferential treatment from insulin. Increased insulin tells your brain to stop eating before you run out of the limited storage space in your muscles and liver for glucose. Think of this storage space as a closet in your house. You know, the one you hastily throw stuff in when you have unexpected visitors. Once that space is full, extra energy converts to fat, increasing fatty acids and triglycerides in the bloodstream. Now, carbohydrates are burned for energy instead of fat unless a whole lot of exercise takes place. You can think of the fat storage place as the attic in your house—more room than your closet, and it's pretty rare that you go to the trouble of removing anything you find there!

While insulin also serves as a generalized growth and energy utilization hormone, the hormone known as **leptin** monitors fat levels. It sends powerful messages to the brain to find food and quit expending energy if fat levels are too low. In the earlier scenario of increased fatty acids and triglycerides, leptin tries to inform the brain to stop storing all that fat, but the message gets muted. Even visceral fat around organs can cause leptin resistance, regardless of how skinny you look. The result is insulin resistance and hormone dysfunction. [15]

The stress hormone **cortisol** activates, sending even stronger signals to conserve energy through these perilous times. As you can see, a vicious feedback loop emerges of metabolic hormones frantically sending the exact wrong messages to your brain, no matter how much you've eaten or how full you should feel. By this point in my earlier analogy, you're moving all your important furniture to the attic and sleeping on the floor!

Obesity is not the root problem. The individual may have an infection, a hormone imbalance, or a food sensitivity and the only way to find out is to ask the right questions. "How can I lose weight?" might only address a symptom of the true issue. Like an onion, we have to remove the layers of the issue one at a time until we get to the root cause. One of my clients just sent me a picture of himself 50 pounds ago to remind us of how far he's come since we shifted his paradigm to health instead of numbers on a scale.

No one becomes a healthy eater overnight. It takes time to apply new habits and make them sustainable. Have you ever planned to go on a month-long diet, but found yourself in the same old eating habits within a few days? You lacked a foundation of healthy habits to sustain a new dietary framework long term. Transitioning begins at the grocery store and making wise choices before you're hungry. This mindset is needed before you start stocking your pantry. If you're used to the standard American diet, it will take time for your palate to change. For a few weeks, your taste buds will miss the excitotoxins and white sugar that used to fuel you, but it's time to change your source of energy. Essentially, you're resetting your system to the way it should react to food.

I worked extensively with a client transitioning to a diet free of gluten, dairy products, and white sugar. After successfully meeting her dietary goals for the week, her deepest craving was for a peanut butter sandwich on white bread. She succumbed to temptation and took one bite, hoping to satisfy her cravings. Sticky chemicals clung to her tongue and teeth, and she spit out that bite, wondering how she had ever stomached those flavors in the past! Her body had already adjusted to eating healthy, and she hasn't tried her former favorite snack since!

The media has benefitted from the confusion about eating healthy because people are continually searching for answers. One sentence taken out of context from research studies can become a popular article or news story. Add politics and advertisers and it's no wonder we had to debunk years of diet mythology about cholesterol, salt, and obesity. Choosing what we eat is the first of many important steps on this natural health path. We'll look a little closer at what a real food diet looks like in a later chapter, but let's first look at some root causes of our health problems.

Action Step: Eat local foods.

Your local farmer is a great place to find fresh food and make long lasting connections.

- Go to eatwild.com or localharvest.org to find local farmers in your area.

- Make the trip a family affair and check out your local farmers market. Everyone can enjoy the experience and pick out their favorites too!

CHAPTER THREE

Real Root Causes

*"We've been to every type of doctor in our area and my child has been on natural supplements, antibiotic medications, and multiple creams, but nothing has worked. Her skin was always breaking out especially around her face. Melanie tested her to find the source of my daughter's problems and discovered food sensitivities and Candida. We put her on a gluten- and dairy-free diet and took herbs for Candida. Her eczema lessened, and once Melanie suggested the **GAPS diet** to heal her gut, it went away completely. Not only did her physical appearance change, but so did her personality. It was like she came out of her shell and felt comfortable in her body for the first time." K.C.*

In this modern medical age, along with distorted perceptions, there are simply too many diagnoses and not enough considerations to solving the problem. Like the client in the testimonial, maybe you're one of the countless parents of children suffering from skin conditions or the millions of women waging war against the bathroom scale. You may be suffering from adrenal fatigue or an athlete trying to decipher the supplement aisles at the vitamin store. We all die, but shouldn't that be after living a long healthy life and not having spent our life savings on medical bills or supplements?

Imagine visiting one physician for most of your life. He or she knew you inside and out and rarely needed to refer you elsewhere.

Targeted prescriptions or therapies eradicated temporary, self-limiting infections and diseases. This acute care model worked well for generations, but it doesn't anymore. It assumes that everyone reacts similarly rather than displaying varied symptoms when health problems occur. That may have been true for chicken pox, but the environment and complexity of issues has changed. Today, protocols and algorithms based on what works for a majority of people increasingly replace the time it takes for a practitioner to really understand individual situations. Knowledge has increased. Specialists thoroughly understand a particular organ or disease. However, seeing the big picture and how our individual genetics interact with chronic illness is beyond conventional medicine. Quality of life is decreasing, costs are escalating, and health care is still trying to match one problem to the corresponding solution and repeat as necessary.

There is a link in a long chain that we have missed that can prevent, heal, and repair our bodies no matter how far gone they are. But I promise it's an easier road back to health than you might think. Let's look a little deeper at the root cause of health challenges we are facing and discover natural treatments based in functional medicine. You may be able to overcome your condition and start living the happy, healthy life of your dreams.

A New Approach

There are two approaches when addressing a health challenge: cover up symptoms with pharmaceuticals or discover and treat the root cause. I'm not implying that medical interventions are always surface level or that a natural remedy automatically transcends symptoms to find causative factors. However, it's easy to forget basic wellness principles when confronted with complex problems.

I had a client who took nasal decongestants daily to keep from getting a sinus infection. The medicine relieved symptoms, but it didn't explain the congestion or provide a long term solution free from side effects. Looking at the functional medicine tree later in the chapter, we can see that there are only a few ways we can become ill or develop symptoms. The cause of the sinus congestion was a dairy sensitivity. Now my client no longer needs to take decongestants because he switched to coconut milk. In this case, we found the root cause and addressed it.

Not everyone's situation is so simple, however. Think of conventional medicine as chopping vegetables with a knife: take an allergy pill and deal with the side effects, but there are no more sniffles. The health philosophies I ascribe to resemble peeling layers off an onion one by one. Food sensitivities as culprits might not be the core layer. Sometimes, solving one issue unveils a previously disguised symptom, and tackling problems out of sequence prolongs healing.

> You can chase symptoms with supplements all day long, but until you get to, and resolve, the root of the problem, you will continue to struggle with your health..

The path to wellness first involves knowing what exactly is causing your symptoms. Wellness isn't a permanent destination; it's a journey. With this new way of looking at health and disease, we realize that there are only a few ways to become sick rather than unique, isolated mechanisms for every named disease. Take irritable bowel syndrome (IBS) as an example. A syndrome is a collection of related symptoms. Instead of simply looking for a name to explain certain symptoms, go deeper to find the cause.

"After running many tests, my last doctor told me I needed to see a psychiatrist because he couldn't find anything wrong with me. I was at the end of my rope and did not want to take any more pharmaceuticals. I couldn't get to sleep or stay asleep. Melanie helped me understand my MTHFR gene defect and directed me to the appropriate lab testing so we could have a better picture of my genes. She walked me through some diet and lifestyle changes that have made the difference in my health. I'm finally sleeping through the night and I feel so much better!" Thomas Kinglsey

Functional Medicine

I use natural health, alternative medicine, and similar terms interchangeably, but functional medicine is a unique modality. It implements cutting-edge medical technology, but shares the practicality and gentle approach appreciated by naturopaths and similar practitioners.

Consider this analogy. Conventional medicine uses a microscope to focus on symptoms in isolation. Complementary alternative medicine implements a telescope as if to see patterns in the stars. Functional medicine can do both. Similar to alternative medicine, functional medicine works from a systems approach. Instead of a straight line between cause and effect, it weaves a web connecting seemingly unrelated factors to solve baffling problems. [16] Without the systematic, focused search for causation functional medicine employs, complementary alternative medicine can be a harmonious but potentially fruitless attempt to alleviate sickness.

Most of the citations in this book are from research studies, because one of the loudest arguments against anything natural or traditional is that it isn't scientific. Academic papers work well to pinpoint the effect of one drug or a function of one organ. Reducing the scope and variables of a study improves accuracy. For results applicable on an individual level and for complex phenomena with multiple variables, the standard approach to research ranges from useless to purposely misguided. Because of this, functional medicine resembles computer modeling for an individual's cancer treatment plan more than easily manipulated research. [17]

The conventional model currently in place standardizes medicine. That's wonderful for standard patients, but not so much for the rest of us. Health problems remain unresolved and providers subscribe bandages such as antibiotics, anti-inflammatories, and painkillers. Those drugs may bring temporary relief but they continue to bury the true problem. There has to be a better way. A way that focuses on optimal lab values for your situation, not whether you are simply in the normal range. A way that looks at nutrition as the central focus to overcoming disease and uses safe, natural herbs and supplements to correct imbalances. I have just described for you functional medicine, a true form of health care.

Functional medicine addresses the underlying causes of disease by shifting the traditional disease-centered focus of medical practice to a more patient centered approach. I like to call it personalized medicine. This technique addresses the whole person, not just an isolated set of symptoms. Instead of seeing your doctor for 10 minutes and having unanswered questions, this new system offers a true partnership with your health care provider. A visit with a functional medicine practitioner is spent discussing your health history and looking at the interactions among genetic, environmental, and lifestyle factors that can influence long-term health and chronic disease. This approach is unique in that it offers the patient an individually tailored health program.

The Root Causes of Illness

Dr. Mark Hyman, a leading functional medicine doctor from the Cleveland Clinic, believes functional medicine is the best-kept secret in science and medicine today. He also believes it can reduce health care costs and improve patient outcomes. How can this be? The diagnoses and treatments of the last century cause errors, waste resources, and focus on expensive management of chronic conditions. [18] Functional medicine compels us to look at health care from a whole new perspective. This patient centered approach allows the practitioner to look past symptoms and undercover real causes to common illnesses. You may be thinking, "There must be a million root causes they'll have to go through to figure out what's wrong with me." Thankfully that's not true. I have outlined below for you the most common causes of diseases. When handled appropriately, the body can heal. I'm living proof of this model.

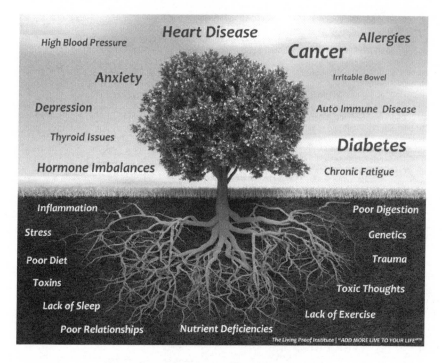

High Blood Pressure

Heart Disease

Cancer

Allergies

Anxiety

Irritable Bowel

Depression

Auto Immune Disease

Thyroid Issues

Diabetes

Hormone Imbalances

Chronic Fatigue

Inflammation

Poor Digestion

Stress

Genetics

Poor Diet

Trauma

Toxins

Toxic Thoughts

Lack of Sleep

Lack of Exercise

Poor Relationships

Nutrient Deficiencies

The Living Proof Institute | "ADD MORE LIVE TO YOUR LIFE"™

It's All About Our Cells

We have trillions of cells organized into tissues and organ systems allowing us to move, breathe, think, and eat. They secrete and accept countless substances that affect how they function. Cells need a variety of nutrients to grow and fight disease. When cells malfunction the body is no longer able to maintain homeostasis (balance) by regulating and repairing itself. All we have to do for our health is give our cells what they need and protect them from what they don't need. When a health challenge is present, either cells lack necessary substances or a toxic substance affects cells and tissues. Cellular deficiency and toxicity are the two causes of disease. Our cells only have a few ways they can become nutrient deficient or toxic. Poor diet, environmental toxicities, and emotional stress, allow inflammation to spread. This can result in the manifestation of symptoms and disease.

Lifestyle choices are the best way to prevent cellular deficiency and toxicity. When we eat nourishing foods, drink mineral rich water, exercise, practice therapies to reduce stress, and use natural medicine appropriately, our bodies will be free from disease. Similar to a flourishing plant with enough sunlight, water, and good soil, the body knows how to take care of itself, provided it has what it needs to do so. But as we will see next, there are several pathways that lead away from vibrant health and to disease.

Environmental Stress (Toxins in the Environment)

We are barraged with toxins every day. It requires a conscious choice to be toxin free. Parabens, pesticides, heavy metals, food colors, food preservatives, medications, air and water pollution, chlorine, and plastics are just some of the toxins we come in contact with every day. In fact, the average person contacts over a hundred chemicals a day. Consider that companies only have to show that each chemical is relatively safe in isolation and in limited doses. The laws governing product safety haven't been updated for a generation. Small toxic exposures each day will increasingly exceed our ability to detoxify. [19]

"Five toxic trace metals: antimony, beryllium, cadmium, lead, and mercury are involved in at least half of the deaths in the US and much of the disabling disease." Henry Shroeder, MD, from **The Poisons Around Us.**

A growing body of research links toxins to a wide variety of symptoms and syndromes such as rashes, behavioral and mental problems, and gastrointestinal disorders. Low level exposures to certain chemicals disrupt hormones, resulting in serious problems that range from infertility to cancers that rarely existed a century ago. These diseases are difficult to diagnose and cure using a conventional medical approach and cost $210 billion annually. [20, 21]

Almost a billion pounds of pesticides are dumped into the environment every year. [22] Purchasing or growing organic food is one way to limit exposure to pesticides. Food storage also becomes an issue, as most containers are plastic and coated in **BPA**, a synthetic compound we'll discuss more in the water chapter. Choosing glass or stainless steel to store food is a much safer option. We don't often think about the clutter in our garage, but usually there is a whole host of chemicals we potentially could come in contact with every day.

Genetics

One of the most manipulated terms in conversations about health is the word, "genetic". We've been led to believe that genes control health directly. Rather, the environment we create for our cells controls the expression of our genes. True genetic diseases exist today but affect less than five to 10% of the population. [23] What we do have control over is our environment, which has changed much more rapidly in the last few generations than our genetic material has.

> "Genetics loads the gun and environment pulls the trigger," says Dr. Soania-Mathur.

"Genetics loads the gun and environment pulls the trigger," says Dr. Soania-Mathur. [24] Despite Dr. Soania Mathur's diagnosis of Parkinson's, she still works as a medical doctor. Rather than accepting our genetic fate, remember that genes are often triggered by lifestyle-dependent environmental factors. Genetic testing from 23andMe.com or similar inexpensive services provides raw data on your genetic predispositions, which you can then submit to other websites such as MTHFR.net or LiveWello.com to see your risk factors for certain conditions. Remember that nothing is inevitable. Genes are simply the blueprint for life that instructs our bodies how to develop from one cell into an entire human. About one quarter of our genes express (turn on) automatically to determine attributes such as hair color. Similar to a computer, most of the other genes are coded instructions that sit dormant until activated. Most genes require some sort of trigger, usually emotional or environmental, in order to express themselves.

What about health problems that "run in the family?" Think of a genetic predisposition to disease as a weak link in a chain—a weak link with the potential to break, but only if excessively stressed. By enhancing function of cells, genetic predispositions can remain potential problems, rather than becoming real problems regardless of what runs in the family. Having a genetic mutation predisposes you to some conditions, so it's best to get tested to determine what further steps need to be taken. We all have highly individualized liver enzymes (part of **liver metabolism**), which is why some people react so differently to certain supplements or drugs. Toward the end of this book, we'll look at studies showing that even our emotions have the ability to turn genes on and off.

The most common genetic variation I see in my practice is with **MTHFR**, a single nucleotide polymorphism (**SNP**). MTHFR regulates methylation and folate. The function of MTHFR is reduced in affected individuals, causing a wide range of side effects from liver detoxification symptoms to clotting disorders. Because MTHFR makes it difficult to process certain nutrients, managing it requires a holistic approach. One of the leading experts and educators on this topic is Dr. Ben Lynch, who hosts MTHFR.net. Primarily, those affected can control the genetic manifestations with lifestyle changes, diet choices, and supplements.

Infections and Immune Challenges

Bacteria, viruses, parasites, candida, and other invaders can have long-term effects if not dealt with properly. As these invaders weaken the immune system, our body doesn't know what to react to anymore, causing food sensitivities and nutritional deficiencies. This cycle repeats over and over, burying the original infection or issue under a slew of seemingly unrelated symptoms. You can have more than one infection present at one time, for example someone may have the **Epstein-Barr virus**, H. Pylori, and a staph infection.

We often think of parasites as giant hungry worms, but most are tiny organisms that disrupt the balance of beneficial bacteria in our bodies. The spirochetes of Lyme disease are difficult to spot even with a microscope. Parasitic invaders poison the body as they steal nutrients and excrete toxins. Low energy is a major complaint, which makes sense since parasites are the equivalent of hungry, sloppy house guests who won't leave.

Almost 33% of the population has been exposed to the top five parasites in the US. You don't have to travel the world to get a parasite, they are readily available right here from food, household pets, and a multitude of insects. Because of parasites, even owning a cat increases the risk of contracting schizophrenia. Parasitic infections are difficult to diagnose via Western medical models. If test results show Lyme disease, there are usually co-infections that need to be treated as well. Beyond digestive problems, parasites cause heart failure, blindness, birth defects, mental illness, and death. [25, 26]

Candida seems to be a bit of a buzz word these days and for good reason. With the consumption of processed carbs and sugars at an all-time high, this naturally occurring fungus in our gut is loving it and deciding to take over. Candida crowds out beneficial bacteria, weakening our defenses when we come in contact with other harmful pathogens. We become prone to harmful infections causing fatigue, digestion issues, skin problems, sugar and carbohydrate cravings, and even emotional problems manifested as ADHD, anxiety, or depression. Whatever names our symptoms answer to, the key is that many of them are associated with infection.

> Most of my clients have had infections for quite some time and come to me having been diagnosed with chronic fatigue, psoriasis, eczema, other skin issues, or fibromyalgia. Other problems triggered by infections are severe seasonal allergies or **autoimmune diseases**, such as Hashimoto's thyroiditis, rheumatoid arthritis, ulcerative colitis, and lupus.

Many people are walking around with low-grade infections that can be resolved by following functional medicine guidelines. First it's important to know which infections you have. This can be done via blood, stool, or even **muscle testing**. You will likely need to find a natural or functional medicine doctor to help with these tests. When I was hospitalized for my heart condition years ago, doctors did everything they knew to find the root cause, but they weren't able to determine that I had a severe parasite infection. It may take time, but the body is strong and can recover from such infections.

Emotions (Beliefs, Attitudes, Emotional Trauma)

Negative or unexpressed emotions can cause just as much stress to our body as an immune invader or food sensitivity. They can interfere with organ function and cause unnecessary stress on the body. Cover up core issues and imbalances with supplements, pharmaceuticals, or therapies all you want, but until we deal with underlying causes, the body finds a way of manifesting them. Emotions do not simply vanish, they must be processed and dealt with. **Emotional release work** is a tool we will discuss further and is a much easier alternative than a full body MRI scan for what could be psychosomatic symptoms.

Food Sensitivities and Nutritional Deficiencies

Our digestive system doesn't simply digest and eliminate food. Our microbiome is home to billions of microbes that live in or on our bodies. Most of them live in the intestines. These microbes influence immunity, mental health, emotions, detoxification, and hormones. The lining of our gut separates food and this wonderful collection of germs from our immune system. This usually prevents food sensitivities, inflammatory conditions, and chronic diseases. Tight junctions between the cells lining the gut are naturally permeable to nutrients and other selective small molecules.

> We are not always what we eat; we are what we digest and assimilate.

Damage to the lining of the gut can present itself as digestive problems, poor nutrient absorption, and food sensitivities. Diarrhea and constipation prevent nutrients from proper absorption. Think of an assembly line that suddenly changes speed. The finished product isn't going to look right. Chronic exposure to foods and medications that irritate the gut wall weaken the ability to absorb nutrients. We are not always what we eat; we are what we digest and assimilate.

A food sensitivity occurs when a microscopic particle of food sneaks between the tight junctions and out of your gut to the bloodstream. When the immune system sees a foreign particle of undigested food, it assumes the rogue particle is an invader and sounds the alarm whenever those undigested food particles resurface. This is what we call "**leaky gut syndrome**" or "permeable gut." Leaky gut is caused by stress, nutrient deficiency, antibiotic use, birth control pills, and eating improperly prepared, indigestible food. [27]

Core Dysfunctions and Imbalances

Inflammation

When root causes aren't addressed, core dysfunctions develop. Inflammation shows us two distinct truths I learned during my functional medicine training: that many factors result in one condition and that one factor can cause unrelated conditions. Most people associate inflammation with sprained ankles or achy joints, but inflammation is a natural response to any foreign invader in our body. Inflammation is first and foremost a health maintenance process. Inflammation cannot be measured directly by a single lab test but rather is viewed through many different parameters. Inflammation has four important wellness responsibilities: it repairs tissue, kills all types of invading microbes, eliminates toxins, and kills cancer cells. The problem occurs when inflammation becomes chronic and systemic instead of localized and restorative.

"It's not about calories in, calories out. It's about lowering inflammation, and gluten, sugar and dairy increases inflammation in your body." – Erica Kasuli

Chronic inflammation is present in every disease. It can be similar to an overzealous 911 operator. To clear the roadway for a simple fender bender she dispatches a few police cars, an ambulance, and a couple of fire trucks. Eventually there are so many emergency vehicles that traffic is disrupted and certain streets can become closed. Comparably chronic and out-of-control inflammation spreads and increasingly disrupts bodily functions.

To handle inflammation in our systems, we need a simple ratio of roughly 3:1 Omega-3s to Omega-6s, but current American diets skew that balance to 20:1. **Omega-3 fatty acids** decrease rates of mental illness, cancer, heart disease, and a host of other problems. [28]

You might be wondering why all this information matters since the redness and pain of inflammation tends to eventually resolve. However, as chronic inflammation develops, your immune system starts spending most of its time on red alert. How hard would it be for you to work at a place with fire alarms going off continually and the sprinkler system activating every time someone lit a scented candle? In the process of extinguishing that little flame, a lot of innocent people and office furniture are going to get soaked. That's how chronic inflammation works. At first you might not be able to tell from the outside of the office building that anything is abnormal. This is why we need to pay close attention to what our bodies are telling us. If we keep treating that recurring sinus or urinary tract infection with antibiotics and covering up every twinge with pain relievers, our bodies never fully get to complete the last step in the inflammatory response: healing. In other words, you might take inflammation more seriously if I refer to it as arthritis, lupus, colitis, diabetes, cancer, Alzheimer's, or heart disease.

Autoimmune Issues

Imagine an army firing missiles at a radar blip in their territory that turned out to be a large bird instead of a stealth bomber. During that distraction, a real enemy would find it easier to invade. In the body, confusion often begins with a leaky gut allowing food proteins to encounter the immune system. Pathogens such as viruses, parasites, and Candida take up residence as inflammation becomes systemic. The immune system can no longer quickly detect the difference between friend or foe, foreign invaders or healthy tissues.

It starts reacting to proteins in the food you eat and the air you inhale. Asthma, rheumatoid arthritis, type 1 diabetes, Hashimoto's, and multiple sclerosis are examples of autoimmune disorders that likely began with an inflammatory response to a foreign invader. That foreign invader could have been an undigested food protein, an infection such as mold or a virus, dust, or even a chemical such as food dyes. Using our previous example, food sensitivities and an infection can trigger IBS—the gut lining is damaged and permeable and the person usually lacks adequate beneficial bacteria.

Physician and professor Dr. Terry Wahls said she recently overcame her diagnosis of advanced multiple sclerosis by following the paleo diet and healing her gut. Research shows that inflammatory compounds that affect the brain and muscle memory decrease with the high fat and protein and low carbohydrate foods that such a diet provides. [29, 30] Those suffering from an autoimmune disease can work on healing the gut by following the GAPS, **Paleo Autoimmune Protocol**, or Specific Carbohydrate Diet; you can find out more about these in the Glossary and later this chapter. While healing the gut, work with a qualified practitioner to get rid of chronic or low grade infections. In this population, heavy metal toxicity often needs to be addressed.

Impaired Detoxification

If we can't detox properly, even the healthiest diet won't be enough to resolve our symptoms. The main detoxification organ is the liver. Its primary job is to convert toxins, most of which are fat-soluble, into water soluble compounds for elimination. But there's so much more to detoxification than the liver. Impaired detoxification from **toxic burden**, **methylation defects** like MTHFR, or other causes can result in hormone imbalances, skin problems, brain fog, mood disorders, and low energy. Our liver has three main phases of detoxification: transformation, conjugation, and transportation. It's a complex process involving hundreds of enzymes and genes with significant individual differences.

I'll describe the stages of liver detoxification in the context of cleaning house. First, collect all the trash from every room in the house and put it in the garbage can outside. You then take the can to the curb. Lastly, you wait for the garbage man to remove the garbage. If any of the steps are stalled, you will have a buildup of garbage (toxins) in your house (body). Since bile empties metabolized chemicals into the intestines for elimination via the kidneys, even an all-star liver can't do its job without a supporting cast. [31]

By now, you know I'm all about listening to your body. But, sometimes it can be difficult to decipher what the problem is from symptoms alone. This is where functional lab tests prove useful.

Tests with Answers

We've established that there are only a few causes to many different symptoms. Naming diseases doesn't give us any insight into how to care for you as a whole to eradicate the symptoms. Functional medicine offers unique lab testing that allows us to see a clearer picture of what occurs on a biochemical and cellular level. Before continuing the journey, it's time to really get to know what is going on inside of you.

The best way to do that is to cut yourself open from head to toe and take a good look. Just kidding! I propose simple and safe alternatives to provide the needed knowledge. It's important to note that many of these tests (including blood work) can be obtained on your own. Have a practitioner assess your results and create the best possible program for you. Most of them require someone highly trained in functional medicine as the answers lie in "optimal" results rather than merely "normal." Knowledge is power. Once I knew what was causing all the damage in my body, a straight path to health appeared. I stayed focused on the root causes, and you can too. Yes, I had inflamma-

> "Food is to your body what gas is to your car. After meals you should feel energized, happy, confident and ready to take on the day. If you are feeling bloated, tired, exhausted, drowsy, depressed; change fuel."
> – Erica Kasuli

tion from infections, food sensitivities, heavy metals, and mineral imbalances. But I didn't know that until I got tested to determine exactly what was going on. Below are some tests I recommend:

Saliva Hormone Testing:

Bio-Health Laboratories has a few different testing options, but one test I run on almost all my clients is their adrenal hormone panel.

The 201 test is great for measuring the adrenal hormone cortisol for men and women, and the 207 measures estrogen and progesterone throughout a woman's cycle. Most functional medicine doctors will routinely check hormones via saliva.

Blood Testing:

You can always ask your doctor to run specific blood work panels, but I often find it easier and quicker to use mymedlab.com. You can order the test you want and bring the results with you at your next appointment so your physician or alternative health care practitioner can go over the results with you. For thyroid patients, I often recommend looking into the website and book by Janie Bowthorpe, *Stop the Thyroid Madness*. She provides information on the necessary testing to determine what is going on with your thyroid and its hormones. Also, I recommend the Spectra cell blood test for testing minerals and micronutrients. This test can be ordered through mymedlab.com or at Any Lab Test Now locations.

Hair Mineral Analysis Testing:

This is a test that uses hair to determine mineral status. It measures deficiencies to determine if you need more zinc, chromium, or other minerals. Hair mineral testing helps determine which specific minerals should be added to the diet or which ones to further supplement.

Stool Testing:

There are two **stool testing** labs that create a good combo to know if infections attack the gut. They test the samples by searching for infectious agents or screening for genetic material. The Biohealth #401H Stool Test is recommended along with the Metametrix Genova Lab GI Effects Stool Test. I've found that comparing the results from both tests gives me a broad yet detailed picture of infectious organisms and digestive problems.

Doctor's Data Heavy Metal Testing:

This is a urine test to determine heavy metals. Heavy metal toxicity is a serious problem but manifests as vague symptoms that could be mistaken for many of the issues we've already talked about.

A Natural Path to Wellness

Whether or not you do any testing to determine what is going on inside your body, there are many ways to further improve your health. Below, I have outlined three separate paths depending upon where you are at in your health journey. It's easy to rave about the dangers of environmental pollution and chemicals, but there are practical steps to rid yourself of toxins and avoid acquiring more in the first path, Detoxification. Target autoimmune diseases with a gut healing protocol to take away inflammation's fuel as the second path, gut healing. Lastly, focus on nourishing the body to prevent illness or maintain recovery. After reading each path, you'll likely know which area you need to begin your journey.

After giving nutrition consults and walking people through positive lifestyle changes, I began to notice similarities among my clients whether they had debilitating illnesses or only minor complaints. They came from all walks of life with completely different social, economic, and pathophysiological issues. Despite their varying backgrounds, my clients tend to fit into only one of the three different categories.

Detoxification

It's no surprise that we live in a toxic world. We are bombarded with air pollution, unnecessary medications we take purposefully or ingest

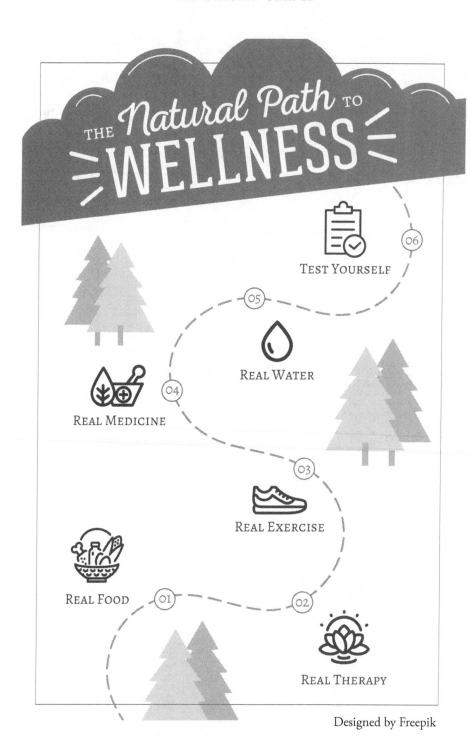

Designed by Freepik

in our tap water as trace contaminants, and chemical additives and preservatives in any food that comes in a box. Detoxification is usually the first step to better health, but what does it mean? Believe me, it's not a random pill you buy off an infomercial at three in the morning. Those shows may look just like your local news, if the headline story was about flushing your colon for six easy payments of $34.31, but be assured that they aren't. Snake oil salesmen are all around us. They might wear suits and spout all the right natural health lingo, or they could dress in long white coats and pretend an abstract research study applies directly to you. The detoxification I'm suggesting involves lifestyle changes that reduce pesticide exposure and chemicals commonly found in processed food and the environment.

Step one in detoxification is to change your diet. This is where you want to begin avoiding white bread, soda (or pop, as they say where I'm from), and white sugar. A detoxifying diet includes large amounts of raw fruits and vegetables to cleanse your cells of toxins you've built up over the years. The principles of food combining are a key part of detoxifying in order to make digestion an easy, low-energy activity so your body can focus on repair. Critics state that the food-specific enzymes and hormones in your digestive system are more than capable of digesting all sorts of food together, and that additives don't present a problem for most people. I give the example of a paper shredder. Just because you can force a credit card and five sheets of paper through it all at once doesn't mean it will have the longevity of a paper shredder you patiently feed one or two sheets of delicate documents at a time. There are many subtleties to food combining, but the one that seems to be the most beneficial is eating fruit on an empty stomach. Try eating fruit 30 minutes before or two hours after a meal. Some seem to benefit from food combining more than others. If your digestion seems off and you are bloated after meals, explore food combining further via the Body Ecology Diet.

It's important to note that a diet based almost completely on raw foods is meant for a short-term cleanse (one or two weeks) rather than a way of life. By strict definition, a food ceases to be raw when live enzymes start dying, usually above 105 degrees Fahrenheit. At the time when I tried it to heal my body, the raw food diet was being portrayed in natural medicine media as the ultimate diet. I noticed diminishing results after a few months and began teaching my clients the value of going raw for limited periods of time. Sure enough, within a few years, raw food advocates such as Daniel Vitalis and Paul Nison came to the same conclusions I did. Safer whole food cleanses I recommend today are the Whole30 Program and the 21-Day Sugar Detox.

Step two involves reducing the toxic chemical load in your environment. Try using non-toxic cleaners in your home. I love using essential oils such as tea tree or Young Living Thieves. It just feels like everything is much cleaner than before, plus it smells great—no more toxic fumes! To be honest though, you don't need anything fancy to clean your home naturally. Equal parts vinegar and water in a spray bottle, some baking soda and a rag and you are set to clean everything spic and span in no time. If you've been around pesticides, hydrocarbons, food dyes, or other chemicals, consider taking the specific homeopathic remedy for the type of toxin affecting you. We will talk more about homeopathics in the real medicine chapter.

It's also time to swap out old chemical-filled makeup and use safer, nontoxic versions. Women are notorious for slathering their faces in petroleum products when the last bit of smoothie in the blender would make a much better facemask than anything in the local spa. **Parabens**, heavy metals, and other chemicals are all found in the makeup and lotion we swear by. It's time to slowly start replacing some of your chemically based or outdated products with paraben free, natural and organic skin care and makeup products. Some of my favorite nontoxic makeup comes from 100% Pure Cosmetics, Coastal Classic Creations, and Jurlique. Remember, you're looking for paraben-free, and read the hopefully short list of ingredients—if it sounds scary, it probably is.

The next thing to do is avoid pesticides. Would you eat an apple sprayed with Raid, wiped off, and then handed to you? I highly doubt it, but there are chemicals stronger than that being poured over our food every day. Glyphosate, a common herbicide found in one of the most popular products on the market, has a whole host of negative side effects, including the estrogenic acceleration of breast cancer. An astonishing amount of people still test for residues of DDT and other toxic pesticides outlawed a generation ago. [32] It's difficult to decipher the combined effects of the scores of pesticides and chemicals that bombard us on a daily basis. One thing we know for sure: eating organic produce and animal products is the best way to limit pesticide exposure. If going 100% organic is not in the budget, stick to the "Clean Fifteen" and avoid the "Dirty Dozen." The lists can be found in the appendix.

Lastly, try to limit your exposure to electromagnetic fields. Health problems associated with **EMF** exposure are difficult to diagnose but include headaches, dizziness, nausea, and disrupted sleep. We encounter EMFs every day from microwaves, cell phones, computers, Wi-Fi, hairdryers, etc. It seems implausible that this invisible energy can be harmful, but thousands of studies collected by the US Library of Medicine and the National Institutes of Health show that electromagnetic sensitivity exists.

So what can we do to protect ourselves? First, limit your exposure to EMF's. Get rid of the microwave and use a battery powered alarm clock to keep electricity out of your bedroom while you sleep. The **Environmental Working Group (EWG)** advises not holding cell phones up to your head, especially for long periods of time. Second, simply take a walk outside barefoot, otherwise known as "**earthing**"; earthing has a grounding effect protecting you from "dirty electricity." Third, you can wear personal protection or buy tools to protect your home and electrical appliances. EnergPolarit makes several wearable diodes to provide personal protection; in fact, I wear a diode necklace every day. You can place diode stickers on your cell phone and connect specific diodes to wall outlets or computers to provide whole room protection from EMFs.

Gut Healing

You've probably heard the old adage that all disease begins in the gut, and I wholeheartedly agree. When a food sensitivity is present, a gut-healing protocol is in order. Special diets are very helpful in healing the gut. The best choice is the one you can stick with. These protocols typically remove difficult-to-digest foods such as grains, dairy, sugar, and other processed foods and introduce healing foods and supplements such as bone broth, cultured vegetables, **L-glutamine**, and zinc.

Two common approaches for chronic digestive or inflammatory issues are the GAPS diet and the **SCD protocol**. The GAPS diet was created by Dr. Natasha Campbell-McBride and focuses on healing the gut, which in turn heals the mind. She reports great success with those on the autism spectrum or those with other neurological disorders. Elaine Gottschall created the Specific Carbohydrate Diet (SCD) and wrote about it in her book, *Breaking the Vicious Cycle*. SCD is geared more towards healing your gut from symptoms such as diarrhea or constipation.

Again, don't just shoot in the dark when it comes to your health. Get tested and find out what's going on first. You may need to complete an anti-Candida herb protocol or a specific parasite cleanse. Key foods for healing your gut are bone broth, healthy fats, and cultured vegetables. How can you tell if you need a gut-healing approach? One clue is if you still have issues after switching to a gluten-free or similar whole-foods diet. For those reacting to a long list of ingredients, the autoimmune paleo diet is an anti-inflammatory approach focused on nutrient dense foods to help heal the body.

Nourishing

Reducing your exposure to toxins and making life easier for your gut is only part of the solution. You will not be at the detoxification level very long and a gut-healing protocol can be usually undertaken in two years or less. This third path maintains wellness. True nourishment comes from re-mineralizing the body with essential nutrients.

Fortifying your diet with adequate amounts of trace minerals is an easy yet overlooked game-changer in so many people's health.

The Weston A. Price way of eating is optimal for maintenance after completing a gut-healing protocol. Think grass-fed beef, pastured butter, organic vegetables, soaked grains, and of course sauerkraut. We'll take a closer look at these nourishing foods in the next chapter. I realize that it is a revolutionary concept that complex health issues can be treated with food where other methods have failed. Food has the power to heal us or hurt us. Every morsel that crosses our lips can either make us healthier or less healthy. What we eat can give us healthy digestion, reduce inflammation, promote a healthy hormone response and keep our minds sharp. It protects our perception of healthy living from the distortions mentioned in the previous chapter. The simplest way to live a nourished life is to eat real food.

**Action Step: Peel the onion
(the layers of your chronic illness)**

1. Get reliable Functional Medicine testing done (Blood Serum, Hormones, GI Tract, etc.).

2. Work with a skilled practitioner who knows how to interpret your results.

3. Create a protocol to fix each of the problems that were found on the tests.

4. After the protocols are finished, retest to make sure you fully restored the body system.

CHAPTER FOUR

Real Food

I'm now able to eat sunflower oil without migraines! I used to get the worst migraines from anything with nuts or seeds in them. Thank you, Melanie!" Jeanine Misch

In the midst of my sickness, I knew food would be an integral part of my healing process. I had no idea studying the work of a dentist who practiced over 50 years ago would have such an impact

> "Life in all its splendor is Mother Nature obeyed."
> –Weston A. Price, DDS

on my life and health. Studying traditional people groups like the Mali changed my perspective on food forever.

To say Dr. Price's studies changed my life would be an understatement. His work has shaped my beliefs on food and nutrition not simply because of what he wrote, but when I applied the principles he found to my own diet, I saw dramatic improvements in my health. At the time I was reading Dr. Price's book I was caught up in the raw food movement. I wasn't seeing improvements in my health even though I was eating a primarily raw, plant based diet. Unfortunately, the raw food movement's main component also became their greatest flaw, the idea that constantly cleansing the body is the only way to true health. I remained faithful to the diet until I could not eat another heavy, nut-based meal. It was then that I found the traditional food movement—out with my raw blender soups and in with homemade stock, slow-roasted meats, and cultured veggies! I became a new person.

So who was Dr. Price and what did he discover in his research? What are the healthiest foods to consume each day? Let's discover together what nourishing whole foods really are. We'll dive into raw milk, nourishing animal foods, plant-based foods, and learn the art of fermenting foods.

Pioneering Research in Nutrition and Health

Dr. Weston A. Price was a well-known and respected dentist in Cleveland, Ohio. He served as the head of research for the National Dental Association. Over time, Dr. Price became concerned about the increasing number of dental deformities (i.e., crooked and crowded teeth) and poor health in his patients, especially children. He became intrigued by reports about isolated, non-industrialized peoples with beautiful teeth and seemingly stellar health. [33]

In the early 1930s, Dr. Price began traveling the world studying traditional peoples and their diets. "Traditional" can also mean "primitive," but for our purposes more accurately describes a culture existing on real foods in their original form passed on from generation to generation. In the course of more than 10 years, his research took him to isolated Swiss villages, African tribes, and many other places and cultures. Though the diets varied widely from culture to culture, Dr. Price consistently found straight teeth without decay, good physiques, high fertility, longevity, and resistance to disease among the peoples who only ate their traditional diets.

For example, in the Loetschental Valley of Switzerland, villages existed that were untouched by modern foods or even basic technology such as pasteurization. From their cows eating lush grass, the villagers embraced butter, milk, cheese, and cream. The villagers also ate a dense, sourdough rye bread and occasionally had meat and the few vegetables able to grow at high elevation during the short Swiss summers. This was in stark contrast to villages just outside the valley.

There, people turned away from the traditional Swiss diet in favor of eating processed and refined foods such as white flour, jam, canned foods, condensed milk, and white sugar.

Those eating a modern "civilized" diet showed signs of crooked, decaying teeth and suffered from degenerative modern diseases previously unseen in these communities. Dr. Price used unique methods to document the health differences between communities. He contacted local health boards for records and statistics and would line up entire villages for examinations. Besides assessing villagers for tooth and facial deformities, Dr. Price performed thorough physical examinations and transported local food to his laboratory for microscopic and chemical inspection. [33]

Dr. Price chronicled the results of his inspections in his sentinel work, *Nutrition and Physical Degeneration*. His laboratory research showed that traditional diets contained vastly more concentrated amounts of vitamins and minerals compared to the American diet of his day. Traditional diets provided four times the water-soluble vitamins and minerals, and at least 10 times the fat-soluble vitamins. [33] Surprisingly, the main source of these storable vitamins was from animal foods such as butter, fish eggs, shellfish, organ meats, eggs and animal fats. Traditional people groups instinctively favored foods rich in the fat soluble vitamins A and D and saved them in famines as "sacred" foods to ensure healthy future generations. They are vital to our health because, in their natural form, these two vitamins act as catalysts for mineral absorption and protein utilization. Modern science has known this for years, but artificially fortified vitamin A and D milk from the grocery store has yet to make a dent in osteoporosis rates.

So should we start booking flights to Switzerland? In our modern lives, there must be an easier way to apply Dr. Price's findings than living in a remote village. Before I show you how to find these traditional foods and easily make them in your own kitchen, let's explore why this isn't another fad or superfood of the month diet.

Diet of the Month

We need to reclaim our health with optimal food choices. Unfortunately, we are bombarded with words like these every day:

Calories	Metabolism	Special K
Fat	High-protein	The food pyramid (My plate)
Protein	Low-calorie	Low-fat
Carbohydrates	Skim milk	No-fat
Low-carb	Vegan	Diet soda
Aspartame	Vegetarian	Sugar-free
High-carb	Whole-wheat	Soy milk

I'll make one exception for "counting calories." How is it possible to enjoy eating when you begin a meal with math?

We've created a monster—a false nutrition monster eating fortified snack cakes and drinking zero-calorie soda moving at lightning speed that won't be slowing down unless we hit the brakes. It is a waste of time to go through the positive (but mostly negative) accolades for the above nutrition buzzwords. I'll make one exception for "counting calories." How is it possible to enjoy eating when you begin a meal with math? Judging a food only by its calorie content is like filling up your gas tank with whatever will provide the most combustion. Gasoline, liquid oxygen, and hydrogen are all wonderful propellants, but only one of them belongs in your car. What we eat far outpaces every other influence on our wellness.

This one step is an important principle which lays the foundation for a new you: eat real food. It seems so easy, right? Unfortunately, fake food pretending to be real food is lining aisle after aisle of our supermarkets and does not promote health in our hormones, our digestion, our brain, or our inflammatory response. This includes foods packaged with long lists of ingredients: anything made with white flour, fast food, and genetically modified foods. What we put in our mouths has the power to either nourish or harm us. Simply knowing information on which foods are healthy doesn't always mean we make the best choices. Even choosing healthy foods can get complicated; otherwise, I'd print you out a shopping guide and send you on your way to the grocery store. We have emotional connections with food which need resolved as well as physiological connections. That's why you might be craving a particular item right now.

> *"I have dealt with digestive issues for at least the last 20 years. I never felt comfortable after I ate a meal and always had the urge to go to the bathroom. I ate very healthy (no processed food or white sugar, very little dairy, and only ate whole grains) and yet I still had these issues. I met with Melanie and had Nutrition Response Testing done. After following the guidelines and avoiding the foods my system was sensitive to, I began to feel better within a week. I can testify that today I am completely free of my symptoms. Praise God and thank you Melanie." Kathy Kappela*

I'm going to show you my views on food and the research studies and conclusions that form the basis of my findings and give you testimonials demonstrating the healing power that can take place in a body given the appropriate foods. Through my trials and tribulations in finding out what worked for me as well as helping others, I realized there were many paths to wellness through food. For example, some do better with more protein while others do better with more carbs. Just because a food is considered healthy does not mean it's the food for you, and that's okay. Learning what foods work for you is a process. What makes this type of information so special? You will never question whether anything you put on your plate is healthy or not because you will be empowered to make educated food choices for as long as you live.

	Standard American Diet	Highly Nourishing Diet for Comparison (using organic foods)
Breakfast	Cereal and milk	Scrambled pastured eggs with spinach cooked in pasteurized butter
Snack	Granola bar	Soaked nuts and seeds
Lunch	Ham sandwich	Rice noodles with stir-fried veggies and chicken
Snack	Cheese curls and soda	Bananas and figs or avocados and olives
Dinner	Frozen pizza	Homemade bone broth soup, lots of cooked veggies topped with sauerkraut

Seems so harmless, but when we break it down the Standard American Diet is severely nutrient deficient. When I look at the left menu I see high-gluten wheat, sugar, high-fructose corn syrup, hydrogenated (poisonous) fats, pesticides, GMOs, hormones, and food preservatives.

The Standard American Diet will fill your belly but it will leave you highly malnourished. The highly nourishing menu also on the chart will make a world of difference in your health. It may take time and it will definitely be a journey, but food is the foundation for a healthy life.

"I had suffered from tension headaches and migraines for years. In the 1990's, I tested the effects of red wine, chocolate, aged cheeses, MSG, etc. I noticed no correlation between these things in my diet and my headaches. In 2013, my doctor recommended the film Fat, Sick, and Nearly Dead. *I watched it and started*

juicing. I began to think my headaches were more related to my diet than I had previously thought. I started eating ancient grains, instead of just whole wheat. I also started consuming more organic products, including milk. Between these changes and juicing, my headaches were only slightly reduced. Then, I met Melanie. She discovered things going on in my body no one had been aware of. She had me eliminate gluten, dairy, and refined sugar. This was difficult for me at first, but not nearly as hard as I had thought it would be. With Melanie's supplements and recommendations, my migraines and tension headaches have greatly reduced in number and severity. For someone who had headaches about 6 -7 days per week, this is HUGE! I also have more energy." Jane Desoi

Raw Milk

We'll start our quest for real food with the most controversial. If you want some easy entertainment, type "raw milk" into the YouTube search bar and prepare yourself for an onslaught of ridiculousness. You might understandably be incredulous about a food revered as manna from heaven or poison from that other place.

Our story begins with a distillery during the Industrial Revolution. Job seekers left their rural farms for the cities and brought with them a greater demand for raw milk and fermented beverages. Trying to capitalize on both, the novel idea emerged of bringing cows into the cities and confining them next to the distilleries where they were fed "hot, reeking swill," the byproducts from making whiskey. Unfortunately, the resulting milk was more toxic than the alcohol. The animals were treated so poorly that their milk lacked nutrients and was poisonous regardless of its use.

After public outcry, officials increased the availability of clean raw milk and created subsidies to pasteurize the cheap, yet toxic, milk. Infant mortality decreased and everyone was happy, for a while. [34] Raw milk was banned after fictitious magazine articles surfaced linking raw milk to fevers, vague symptoms, and diseases similar to tuberculosis. [35] Interestingly enough, when Dr. Price visited places that shared this fear, the cases of tuberculosis all occurred in the modern villages drinking pasteurized milk and eating processed foods. [36] The latest analysis of raw milk studies further clarifies the issue of safety, although the significance of vitamins and enzymes destroyed by pasteurization is still controversial. What is becoming widely accepted is that raw milk decreases the incidence of allergies and lactose intolerance. It does not increase the risk of cancer or disease. [37] We can conclude that part of the controversy is because, generally speaking, milk quality is variable enough to meet any of the wild claims we've discussed thus far.

Pasteurization May Not Be the Answer.

On the low end of quality is factory-farmed cow's milk that must be pasteurized (heated almost to the point of sterilization) for any human consumption. Similar to the "distillery cows" of the Industrial Revolution, most of the dairy herds in this country are deprived of exercise and sunlight and confined to narrow stalls. Instead of a natural diet of green plants, the cows are fed grains, food and animal waste, candy, hormones, and antibiotics. After the milk is pumped from these poor cows, it needs to be pasteurized, homogenized, and fortified before it can be poured into jugs and cartons and accepted as a reasonable beverage. [38]

Don't get me wrong; when Louis Pasteur discovered pasteurization in the mid-1800s, he made a major breakthrough in disease prevention. However, the high temperatures required to kill germs also make milk harder to digest by denaturing proteins and their enzymes. Is it any wonder that so many of us can't tolerate conventional dairy products? Some of my clients who are lactose intolerant can actually tolerate raw milk, much to their surprise.

One of the most ardent defenders of raw milk is Mark McAfee, raw milk production expert and founder of Organic Pastures Dairy. I interviewed him for a fresh and current perspective and he had this to say:

"A century-long war against bacteria and raw milk has drawn to a close with a fiercely fought re-emergence of raw milk in the market place. After 100 years of pasteurizing milk with ever increasing temperatures, finally the consumer's gut could not take it anymore. Dollar voting from that same consumer's wallet has abandoned milk for other non-milks or juices. Now, the FDA has created the most allergenic food in America. Yes, number one. Pasteurized milk is also the origin of lactose intolerance in 30 percent of the population. We must all remember that pasteurized milk is a friend of shelf life and warehouses and not your GUT. Feed the gut and feed the very basis of health."

Referring to the science of raw milk, Mr. McAfee added:

"According to Dr. Bruce German, PhD at UC Davis Milk Genomics research lab, pasteurized milk is not digestible by children. As we go forward, look to the [$3.5 billion] NIH funded Human Genome project and its discovery that bacteria are what make us a complete human. When our bacteria are missing, humans become a sickly autoimmune mess. Mankind must wake up quick or fall into a deep sleep to never awaken. Food drives our health…not the frequency of visits to the doctor's office or the number of pills we take."

Call the SWAT Team.

You probably sense a pattern in the foods I am promoting and the great contrast between a healthy cow providing milk or beef and a sick one that provided the hamburger patty for your fast food meal. Most people reading this book can attest to not feeling well after fast food, but dairy experiences are more individualized. My first experience with raw milk involved pulling up to a strange house and letting myself into their garage. As instructed, I gingerly opened the refrigerator located between a car and some empty egg cartons and found the stash. I placed my money in the envelope and hurried to my car, my fist clenched around a cold gallon of raw milk.

Actually, sneaking around a stranger's house while their Siberian husky growled at me was the easy part. My husband and I had to sign contracts, waivers, and split "ownership" of a random Amish herd of cows in the middle of nowhere that we occasionally had to visit. It's probably easier to obtain crack than raw milk.

I poured a glass of milk as soon as we got home, half expecting to hear a SWAT team helicopter or a sudden knock at the door. It tasted better than regular milk, but I wasn't magically transformed into a routine milk drinker. I finished the glass, but what was I going to do with the rest of the gallon and my complimentary quart of cream?

Cultured Dairy

There in my kitchen, milk mustache intact, I suddenly remembered a passage from Jordan Rubin's book *The Maker's Diet.* He mentioned that cultures throughout the world fermented milk products using techniques similar to making wine or sourdough bread. The results are loaded with healthy bacteria, don't easily spoil, and have little in common with today's cheeses and yogurts. B vitamins and calcium levels are already much higher in the milk of properly-cared-for cows and only increase as the milk ferments. [39]

We mostly know fermented milk as yogurt. Unfortunately, commercial yogurt is fermented for four hours or less, not giving the beneficial bacteria enough time to actually ferment the milk. Then, of course, sugar and fillers are added to make the product seem like it has truly soured. Kefir is another fermented milk choice with benefits that are pretty much astounding. Making cultured milk couldn't be easier if you're up for it, but most areas have local farmers who sell homemade raw milk yogurt and homemade kefir. Choose your preference, but remember that milk is always best cultured.

My last words on milk are as follows. Raw milk from grass-fed healthy cows is best. It's even better when fermented and made into yogurt, cheese, or kefir teeming with probiotics. BUT, raw milk is not going to save the world or any and all of your health problems. Some people are still sensitive to dairy products even after following a gut-healing protocol. Your genes sometimes boss you around. We are all different, and our bodies all react in different ways to stress or junk food. That's why my 87-year-old grandpa is healthy as a horse and why I felt the pangs of a heart attack at 21. Paying attention to what our bodies are saying is an important key to health that somehow cleverly got put in the raw milk section. Anyways, trust your body when it doesn't like a food. Milk is a controversial subject, which is why I'm leaving it up to you whether you decide to include it in your diet. Real milk is the only milk I see fit for consumption.

But If I Remove Dairy, What About Calcium?

Removing dairy out of our diet doesn't mean a sudden deficiency in calcium. I've scared many a client when I took their serving of cottage cheese away. But the truth is, most modern dairy products are commercially fortified with artificial calcium which isn't easily absorbed. More often than not, over-supplementation of calcium is becoming a problem as it can decrease levels of other nutrients. Dairy from grass-fed pastured cows has a much higher natural calcium content along with vitamins A and D for easy absorption. In fact, milk or butter won't contain Vitamin K2 unless the cow was organic and grass-fed. [40] If you are worried about your calcium needs, consider eating real cultured dairy, sesame seeds, sardines, dark, leafy greens with butter, and homemade bone broth.

Bones are not just made of calcium. Vitamin C and the minerals magnesium and phosphorus are needed for strong bone development. Two other major players are the fat-soluble vitamins K2 and D3. A low-fat diet makes it more difficult for these factors to channel dietary calcium into bones instead of urine (where they can form spectacular kidney stones). In the short term, calcium apart from these other co-factors is beneficial, but hormones and enzymes redistribute isolated calcium away from the bones to the extent that osteoporosis is worse than before. [40]

The Sensible Carnivore

Okay, so you probably shouldn't pour bone broth over your cereal every morning. Ingesting animal products leads to a balanced approach to disease prevention *or* worsens inflammation and hormone imbalances depending on how the animals were fed and raised. I'm sorry, but there's no room on your plate for factory-farmed chicken or beef. As Americans, we aren't starved for meat. Most people don't need to eat more animal protein but rather need to switch to healthier, more sustainable options incorporating bone broths, organ meats, and pastured eggs. Traditional people groups risked their lives for specific protein foods and fattier cuts of meat for a reason.

> Most people don't need to eat more animal protein but rather need to switch to healthier, more sustainable options incorporating bone broths, organ meats, and pastured eggs.

Protein in its most basic form is the amino acids our bodies use to make and heal soft tissue and the enzymes driving chemical signaling and digestion. Our body cannot create eight essential amino acids, so we acquire them through our diet. Our body, especially organs requiring the most nutrients, depends on amino acids to run smoothly. There are certain animal protein amino acids also available in plant foods, albeit in much smaller quantities. [39] This is why vegetarians include a variety of plant proteins in their diet. For protein needs, opt for whole-food sources of protein. If you need protein fast after a workout or between meals, try Great Lakes Collagen. It dissolves in cold water and improves your overall amino acid profile.

Protein Pretenders

Plant-based proteins and protein powders are all the rage, but they too have their downfall. Brown rice and peas aren't adequate protein sources, and I especially don't recommend soy or any whey from factory farmed cows. Eating soy in its traditional forms such as natto and other fermented soy foods are fine, as I explain in the appendix.

What proteins are Grecian Garden approved? Take a look at the chart below. You have not lived until you've hunted wild beef and eggs. Just kidding.

	Recommended	Not Recommended
Whole-food sources of protein	Organ meats, beef, bison, lamb, chicken, wild caught fish, bone broth, eggs, grass-fed organic whey	Protein powders derived from: brown rice, soy, peas, non- organic or factory-farmed whey.

Organ Meats

By now you've figured out that I don't waste many animal parts when it comes to food, even though buying meat in large quantities from a farm tends to be cheaper than going to the grocery store. But why would anyone eat liver and other organs on purpose? Well, Dr. Price discovered that traditional cultures prized animal heart, liver, adrenal glands, and other organs as "sacred foods" reserved for those trying to conceive or in need of improved health. They are the original multi-vitamins. The presence of A, E, and the B vitamins and large amounts of iron and glutathione in organ meats are well documented.

If the idea of eating organ meats leaves you squeamish you can try grass-fed liver capsules. Some of my clients even make their own liver pills by chopping up raw liver into pill sized cubes and freezing it. They pop one of these "pills" each day. We receive vital precursors from organ meats. One example is choline, which I often suggest as a supplement to my clients. Choline is a major portion of the neurotransmitter associated with muscle movement and the para-sympathetic nervous system. Choline repairs DNA and incorporates itself into cell membranes. Its role as a liver cleanse is so vital that researchers suggest adding it to parenteral nutrition (intravenous nutrients for patients too sick to digest food through the digestive tract). In the absence of choline, patients experience memory deficits, skeletal muscle abnormalities, and programmed cell death. [41]

Bone Broth

There are some cultures that rely on bone broth as the main source of minerals in their diets. See the previous page for a chart detailing other whole food mineral sources.

Bone broth is rich in minerals like calcium, phosphorus, silicon, magnesium, and sulfur. It also contains trace minerals that are easy for the body to absorb. I like to make a pot of mineral-rich broth on Sunday to have for the entire week. If I have any extra I freeze it. Use it to make extra flavorful rice and quinoa, stir-fried vegetables, and, of course, save it to make soup. A good recipe for bone broth can be found in the recipe section at the end of the book. There is a difference between broth, stock, and bone broth. Of the three, bone broth has the highest mineral content and is generally cooked the longest.

Environmental Concerns

What about the morality of food? Is it right for one person to eat organic and another person to be hungry? It's difficult to find reasonable and wise solutions about this topic. Being a good steward of the environment involves not wasting food (or at least making it into good compost). At our house, it's a terrible tragedy when food silently rots in the back of the fridge before one of us finds and eats it. Despite the local food movement, most of the cost and energy associated with food occurs once you make a purchase and start storing or preparing it. [42]

Cooking your own organic food is still cheaper than fast food, and buying in bulk from a farmer should be no more expensive than the grocery store. If you're opposed to meat for environmental reasons, realize that conventional meat bought from a grocery store and what you could procure from a local organic farmer is totally different. One turns our land into desert, soils our waterways, and fouls our air. However, grass-fed animals are carbon sequesters—unlike a completely plant-based ecosystem.

To better explain the clear alternative to factory farming, I'll use the well-known example from the movie *Food Inc.*, organic farmer Joel Salatin. He maintains that treating individual animals without the respect and honor they deserve is immoral. We have disconnected ourselves from our food supply and from the traditional concept of eating the food most easily grown and raised locally. On his farm, each animal fertilizes, mows, roots, and pecks to create a thriving system not requiring pesticides, antibiotics, or artificial intervention. This way, each animal lives a full, tranquil life, eating the food it enjoys most without fear of predator or imprisonment. [43]

"Out of trillions of organisms that were alive at the beginning of time, are alive now and will be alive at the end of time, only one tampers with its food. You do not want to bet against those kinds of odds." David Wolfe, The Sunfood Diet Success System

Land and Sea Plants

Mom was right—you need to eat your vegetables. Today, that increasingly complex task seems to require a PhD in botany to differentiate nutrient-dense, anti-oxidant rich, pesticide-free plants from their equally leafy imposters. I'm not going to tell you to spit out anything non-organic and that conventional carrots are equivalent to Cheetos. However, just about all of us need to incorporate more vegetables into our diet, so why settle for those grown in depleted soil? Like dairy and meat, plants cannot provide us with nutrients they never received.

As crop yields per acre increase, soil and vegetable quality decrease. Nutrient density is steadily declining. On the cellular level, current agricultural processes grow larger vegetables by increasing the space between cells. Since nutrients are contained in cells, it's like receiving a huge, wrapped gift you tear open to find a little present tucked in a corner of the box. Instead of drawing up nutrients from the roots, factory-farmed plants grow larger and channel photosynthesis to make simple starches and carbohydrates instead of nutrients. That's not the ideal way to lure us away from unhealthier snack options. Besides soil depletion and artificial growing practices, pesticides, and genetic modifications share some of the blame. [44]

Frankenstein-factory-farmed plants incorporate pesticides and other foreign DNA to enhance plant survival and corporate profits. The interaction of these genes with our own is unclear but potentially deadly. I suppose I could quote a couple studies with dying mice to persuade you, but more chilling than those are the accounts of field workers stricken with strange ailments after working in fields where genetically modified fruits and vegetables were planted. [45] Unless a processed food is labeled as organic, it could be genetically modified. I asked my husband about organophosphatides and the newer pesticides and herbicides. As a nurse anesthetist, he deals with nerve poisons and notes that the chemical bonds these pesticides make with our own cells is irreversible.

So how hardy are these plants if they need new DNA, fertilizers, and pesticides just to survive? They wouldn't survive a day in nature because of their low antioxidant content. A plant bred to look good on a supermarket shelf has as much chance in the wild as a guinea pig released into the woods. Wild crafted plants (those found in nature) employ defenses against predators that also serve to increase their nutrient content. Although more research is needed to show the full extent of the effects of genetic modification, there are specific foods of concern.

The list of genetically modified foods is under ten so it can't be that big of a deal, right? Alfalfa, canola, corn, cotton, papaya, soy, sugar beets, zucchini, and yellow squash. Seems pretty easy to avoid. I mean, when was the last time you had a big plate of alfalfa? But check any grocery store right now and try to find one processed ingredient that doesn't have corn. Guess what they are feeding the cow you had for dinner last night? GMO corn, soy, and alfalfa. Rather than investing in recombinant DNA technology detection equipment, eat the organic, nourishing foods I've suggested and it won't be an issue.

As expert forager Daniel Vitalis often says, for all foods always choose the wildest option for nourishment. Heirloom or original varieties of fruits and vegetables haven't had the "rough edges" bred out of them to look prettier longer on a store shelf. I have a section in my garden of edible weeds, and they don't care if I pay attention to them or not. They don't get the watering and compost that my other veggies do, but they thrive on the patch of barren soil where I plant them.

Of course, great food sources aren't limited to what grows out of the ground and grazing animals. Seaweed is an excellent source of minerals, including trace nutrients. It is an abundant source of iodine, to the extent that I once wrote a research paper theorizing its use for hypothyroidism (although I soon discovered it's a surprisingly complex relationship). Learn to make sushi with sprouted rice or cauliflower rice and veggies instead of raw fish. You can also purchase seaweed seasoning from the health food store to season your food. Adding seaweed to cultured vegetables dramatically increases mineral content.

Fish

Fish and fish oil—but not fish sticks—thin the blood to decrease clots, lower blood pressure, and decrease inflammation. The super star of the sea is Omega 3 fatty acid found in salmon, herring, cod, and similar cold water fish. Cod liver oil supports brain and skin development, joint lubrication, retina formation, and may even assist with autism and similar disorders. [39] This brings up the issue of mercury, which is more concentrated in larger fish. However, with the exception of voracious predators that no one in the Western Hemisphere snacks on regularly, fish are rich sources of the nutrient selenium. Along with the herb chlorella, selenium is a potent "mercury muncher" that keeps us free from oxidative damage and the inability to process vitamin C. [46]

Each bite we eat decreases or contributes to inflammation. The precursor to inflammation is in the fats that you eat. You can't eat flax, chia, hemp, or walnuts for your Omega 3's with a poor diet and expect them to convert to the healthy fatty acids EPA and DHA that regulate inflammation. [46] Our modern diets lack the enzymes (Delta 6) dependent on nutrients (vitamins C, B1, B3, B6, and the minerals boron and magnesium) to convert those omegas from ALA to EPA and DHA. Trans fats from margarine and junk food and hydrogenated vegetable oils prevent the necessary conversions even if you pop fish oil supplements all day. If you can't stomach having fish two or three times a week, start remove some of the bad fats from your diet (i.e. shortening and other hydrogenated vegetable oils) and ease fish into your diet by adding Green Pastures Fermented Cod Liver Oil.

Nuts and Seeds

Nuts and seeds are a great source of protein, healthy fat, and minerals but can be difficult to digest if not properly prepared. Soak nuts and seeds before consumption to make them easier to digest and allow our bodies to absorb their nutrients better. It's easy—soak raw nuts and seeds overnight in salt water, then rinse and eat or store in the refrigerator. You can also dehydrate them to be nice and crispy. The soaking process neutralizes enzyme inhibitors, allowing the nuts to be more easily digested. The salt deactivates the enzyme inhibitors and imitates the way the native peoples in Central America treated their nuts and seeds–by soaking them in seawater before dehydrating them.

Think of all the deficiencies in the Standard American Diet. Despite all the multivitamins we pop like breath mints, our enzymes are overworked by the monumental amount of indigestible foods we've consumed day in and day out since birth. We can't extract the nutrients in foods unless we have the necessary enzymes to break down the food we eat. Although in smaller quantities than grains do, unsoaked nuts and seeds contain phytic acid, an anti-nutrient. What does that mean? Phytic acid binds to minerals (calcium, magnesium, zinc, and iron) making it difficult for our bodies to absorb them. [47] Soaking also stimulates the sprouting process (germination), which increases vitamin production to make nuts even healthier.

Grains, Beans, and Legumes

If not properly prepared, grains or grain like seeds can also be difficult to digest and cause a myriad of health problems like insulin resistance, joint pain, and leaky gut syndrome. The problem is that many of these health problems have vague symptoms. I have many of my clients go gluten-free just for a week or two, and often their seasonal allergies or another seemingly unrelated problem disappears completely. This method also highlights the individual approach each person needs to take for their diet, no matter what I or anyone else tries to tell you.

By soaking, sprouting, or fermenting grains (sourdough) and beans first, we are better able to digest the starches properly. To soak, start by adding an acidic medium such as lemon juice, apple cider vinegar, or whey to uncooked grains or beans and immerse in water overnight. Sprouting deactivates phytic acid and increases nutrient availability. Sprouting instructions can be found on the next page. I promise I'm not trying to turn you all into hippies—it's actually common sense. Nuts and seeds need to be eaten by animals to spread and multiply, but this won't happen if the animal manages to digest vital nutrients rather than passing the plant's genetic material unharmed. To get around the plant's natural digestion barriers, animals often store nuts and seeds until they sprout in the ground (or even a seed "soaks" in a chipmunk's cheek). According to Dr. Price, traditional people groups mimicked this behavior to properly prepare beans, grains, nuts, and seeds that were otherwise seen as indigestible. [33] Traditional cultures store these foods in dark, damp, warm, and slightly acidic environments that convince the seed that the time has come to release nutrients and start growing. Even if the resulting product is ground into flour, the nutrients remain because every part of the grain or seed is used and the anti-nutrients were neutralized in the germinating process.

I know you're still thinking about squirrels, so let me use another example. The indigenous Indians of the Americas ground corn into flour, sometimes before any preparation. At some point, they would soak the corn or corn flour in ashes or mineral lime to begin the fermenting process and release B vitamins. The result was a product completely different from the substance used to fatten cattle or make high fructose corn syrup.

To "soak" whole grains/beans/legumes, cover with water and add an acidic medium (a tablespoon of whey, lemon juice, or vinegar) for 12 to 24 hours. Rinse and proceed with cooking. Once you've soaked and rinsed add them back to your mason jar and cover with cheesecloth bound by a rubber band and lay the jar on its side. Rinse the grains two times each day until they sprout–this typically takes two to three days, but you may notice tails poking out after the first day. Remember to keep the jar covered and placed on its side between each rinse. When I first started soaking grains and beans, I would come home from work to my little science experiment taking place in my kitchen. I would rinse my black beans or lentils or brown rice and get so excited when I saw those sprout tails popping through.

I don't want to make it sound like phytic acid is the lone culprit with a food group that the FDA claims should be the foundation of our diet (even if it's a diet surprisingly similar to the one used to fatten cows for slaughter).

Whichever method you choose, it makes these foods easier to digest. In addition to soaking, sprouting also increases nutrients. You can buy sprouted bread, cereal, whole grains, flour, beans, or nuts if you don't have the time to prepare them. Check my resource section in the back of the book for recommended brands.

Since most people do not soak or ferment their grains, many opt to go grain free, or trendier still, paleo. I once bought an expensive wheat free cookie only to realize it still had gluten in it. Although I've been cooking grain free for years, the advantage of the paleo label is that I don't have to scour the ingredients for low quality gluten substitutes. Paleo foods are free from grains, dairy, refined sugar, beans, and other legumes. When I eat beans I soak and sprout them before cooking. I do the same or ferment brown rice, amaranth, and other grain-like seeds. Note that it's not necessary to avoid phytic acid completely; just reduce it as much as possible.

Just a generation ago, wheat had less gluten. Current varieties have been hybridized to contain much more gluten and starch to make extra-fluffy white bread. [48] When I first founded my business, I primarily baked gluten-free food for clients suffering from all the inflammation a grain-rich diet causes. [49]

Fermented Foods

Every traditional people group that Dr. Price studied, fermented part of their food supply. I can remember reading about fermented foods and thinking, "What, leave food out overnight and it's safe to eat? This goes against everything my grandmother taught me." It's true though. The wonder that takes place when we leave foods on counters overnight seems magical. When it's finished fermenting, transfer to the fridge for storage—we've created our own fast food and probiotic condiments. The spicy, salty, sweet additions that make meals special can now come from our own kitchens. These foods have secrets. Tiny, probiotic powerhouses are just waiting to infiltrate our bodies and team up with our immune system to rid of us of bad guys by keeping pathologic bacteria in check. Eating fermented foods along with our meals also has an added benefit of helping us digest what we eat. Sometime we don't always eat the amount of raw foods that we need too, and the addition of cultured vegetables gives us raw living enzymes and probiotics with each and every bite.

Cultured Vegetable Safety

1. Thoroughly wash your hands and the food to be fermented, and use hot water to wash all utensils and equipment. Also, don't ferment strawberries.

2. The salt inhibits harmful bacteria and the spoilage they cause, but if this is your first time you may want to use a starter culture from Body Ecology or Cultures for Health.

3. After culturing, gray, slimy, smelly vegetables should be completely discarded. A jar of bubbly, expanding brine, a yeasty odor, and bright vegetables signal success.

4. If problems persist, consider an anaerobic fermentation jar such as Pickl-It.

You're probably familiar with one cultured food in every grocery store in America: yogurt. Although yogurt has been seen by many as their probiotic savior for a yeast infection, I bring you some not-so-creamy news. Yogurt needs to be prepared traditionally to have any lasting benefits. Just like with properly raised animals producing good meats, and properly prepared grains for our consumption, dairy also needs steps taken to ensure a true probiotic powerhouse with many different strains of beneficial bacteria and yeast. I remember reading about yogurt in Elaine Gottschall's book *Breaking the Vicious Cycle*. She says yogurt is more digestible if allowed to ferment for at least 24 hours. This ensures all lactose is consumed by beneficial bacteria. Check out my website to find a recipe to make 24-hour yogurt with either dairy, coconut, or almond milk (http://tinyurl.com/o9cmmpc is the short link).

Fruits and Sweets

There's a good reason why this section is short. I've already advised you to avoid processed sugars, white flour (Processed wheat is more of a sweet than a grain.), and sweeteners, after all. Especially if you are avoiding unhealthier sweet foods, fruit is a vital, anti-oxidant rich part of a healthy diet. Most vitamin C in supplements is ascorbic acid, but camu camu berries, acerola, and similar fruits provide bio-available whole food vitamin C complexes to provide energy and even fight anemia. You won't find cases of those lining the grocery store shelves because commercial trends favor high-fructose, low-nutrient hybrids that taste very different from wild blueberries or heirloom apples. When scarce, traditional cultures reserved honey, dried fruits, and other natural sweeteners for important occasions.

It was worth traveling to Greece just to reach up and taste raisins and dates perfectly dried by the hot Mediterranean sun. At least once a month I'm baking a gluten- or grain-free dessert sweetened with honey or dried fruit to satisfy my sweet tooth without stumbling along the path to wellness. There are plenty of blogs and recipes with easy instructions, although a beginner might want to use YouTube rather than Pinterest for instructions; gluten-free Pinterest fails can be horrifying. I suggest you try the recipes in the appendix.

What is Real Food?

Food [food] n 1. something that nourishes, sustains, or supplies. Real [ree-uhl, reel] adj 1. true actual; not artificial

In summary, eating real whole foods can have a positive impact on your health and is the foundation for a new you. Try incorporating pastured animal products, cultured vegetables, bone broth, or healthy fats in your diet. I know you'll be feeling better in no time. Next up, let's take a closer look at the water we are drinking.

Action Step: Learn what is really in your food.

- Read the labels of five canned or boxed foods in your pantry.

- If there are chemicals, colors, high fructose corn syrup, or lots of difficult-to-pronounce words, donate them to a local food shelter or compost them.

Action Step: Know the rules.

- Research your state's laws for the sale of raw dairy products. Ask for information from your local dairy farmer or farmer's market.

Raw milk is illegal in some states and in order to get around this, many pasture raised dairy farmers sell their milk as animal feed. That is what occurs in my area of the country. I usually get raw milk, cream, butter, and kefir at our local farmers market. You may be able to get in on a herd share in your area to access raw milk as well.

CHAPTER FIVE

Water: It's not just H$_2$O

At 17 I was put on birth control pills to regulate my period. Little did I know, the underlying issue was PCOS and hormone imbalances. After eight years of being on the pill I started seeing the damage it was doing—vitamin deficiencies, digestive issues, and adrenal fatigue to name a few. After three surgeries to address continued endometriosis problems, I relocated to Pensacola and found Melanie.

After testing, diet changes, natural medicine regimens and the use of essential oils, I did not have to be scared of stopping the pills because I knew Melanie could help me transition without all the side effects I had experienced before. We discussed over hydration as a possible trigger to my interstitial cystitis. Melanie had me add mineral salt to all my water to ensure I was actually hydrating my body. I can't even describe the changes I have seen in myself: digestive issues gone! Energy levels up! Moods balanced! No more frequent urination! The endometriosis pain and acne I had prior to the new treatments has subsided. For the last 9 months I have felt healthier and happier than I have in over a decade, and I'm pregnant! I am more than grateful to finally have the help I have needed all along." Sara Halstead

Water: Do we really need to discuss this? Absolutely. Even something this simple can have a profound positive or negative impact on our health. We'll revisit my water hunting adventure, talk about different types of water, and discuss optimal ways to filter water. I'll even share how to create hydration drinks, as balancing your fluid and electrolyte intake is a key aspect of good health. Despite what you've been told, correct hydration doesn't come from guzzling as much water as possible throughout the day. Some of you will actually need to decrease your water intake; whether you view the glass half empty or half full, let's get started.

Stickers on my Water Bottles

During my sickest times, water would give me a stomachache. That's when you know you have a serious problem, when even a clear mixture of two hydrogen and one oxygen atom doesn't agree with you. I even tried boiling water before I drank it, but nothing helped and my sister was in the same boat. My mom's friend told us we needed to pray over our water before we drank it. She had read the research of Masaru Emoto, the Japanese alternative medicine doctor who claimed that the molecular shape of water is influenced by human prayers and feelings. This is a different person than the photographer who noted microscopic differences between happy and sad tears. Emoto is best known for the beautiful ice crystals he photographed from spring water or formerly polluted water changed by human interaction. We tried something similar by pouring water in a jar, praying, and placing labels on the jar with words like "Health" and "Restoration."

It catapulted me to a new level of lunacy, but my admittedly superstitious actions started the very important process of researching how water and food changed from its natural form before I ingested it. Before that slightly silly experience, I took it for granted that some things would make me sick and that picking out patterns was almost hopeless. I drank an incredible amount of water every day to help flush out whatever toxin was currently making a comfortable home in my system. I believed that favorite proverb of surgeons, usually recited while pouring liters of sterile saline into the abdomen after removing infected gallbladders and such: "The solution to the pollution is dilution." But guzzling all that water in my early days did nothing for my health. Drinking too much water can be just as harmful as drinking too little.

I know what you're thinking: I have water issues. No one else has such a complex relationship with something so simple. Jesus said that he was the bread of life and living water. We talked about sacred food earlier, but water is even more sacred. It symbolizes life and vitality, and in my own culture, water also symbolizes communication because it is still the best method to connect hundreds of rocky islands to the Greek mainland.

I'm certainly not the first person to have problems with tap water. Talk to the millions of Americans who get sick from tap water every year and you'll understand that it has nothing to do with being trendy or enjoying the slightly plastic taste of bottled water. [50] The main point isn't that a milliliter of tap water is a dirty thing, but that if you're sensitive to it you should take every precaution that you can to avoid it. It's hard to underestimate how sensitive someone with autoimmune problems can be to substances that your average person will never have to worry about. The manifestation may show up as a medical diagnosis of eczema, fibromyalgia, or a food and drug allergy. It reminds me of the satirical show *Portlandia*, where "Miss Food Allergy Portland" rode in an ambulance because she was allergic to air, sun, and water.

Different Types of Water

Tap Water

Let's break down the types of water available, starting with tap water, regardless of the original source. The chemicals used to treat water are poisonous, but compared to the rest of the world we still have clean drinking water in the United States. Our sterilized, anti-bacterialized immune systems just can't handle the germ load in most of the world's water. Of course, they also incorporate strong spices in their food to kill bacteria from their water supply. The same food and drink that would send you to the bathroom for days doesn't bother them at all.

I remember entering a new restaurant with my husband and hearing him ask, "Is everyone breaking up with each other in here? Why are they all crying?" I gently reminded him that we were about to eat spicy Indian food and we would look just as melancholy as everyone else once the food affected our tear ducts and sinuses. Ginger and other herbs I recommend for specific infections inhibit bacterial growth in the water supply where these substances are dietary staples. [51]

So now that we know that germ contamination isn't a severe problem with U.S. municipal water, let's discuss where the problem lies (or floats). Of course, if you lived in Toledo, Ohio in 2014, algae and germ contamination were an issue serious enough to warrant a state of emergency. We all can contaminate tap water by simply forgetting to clean faucets and sinks and ignoring clogs that lead to standing water and bacteria formation. Faucet gaskets can release black, oily slime if they break down, and hard water leads to sediment build up if not cleaned appropriately. Lead pipes in older houses are also a problem that must be replaced, just like certain clients with amalgam fillings won't get better until they remove that constant source of heavy metal poisoning. [52]

One of the biggest problems with our water supply is fluoride, which municipalities add to drinking water to strengthen teeth. Ironically, too much fluoride weakens teeth, and the chemical is associated with bone cancer, neurotoxicity, and harmful effects on thyroid and reproductive function. In many municipalities, fluoride is acquired from industrial toxic waste scrubbers that also include radioactive isotopes, lead, arsenic, and other tasty chemicals that the EPA recommends should never exist in our drinking water. Fluoride can cause cardiac arrhythmias and death acutely and osteomalacia (weak bones) chronically. Fluoride also accumulates in the body and stores itself in teeth and bones. [53, 54] Phase out your use of fluoridated toothpaste and water.

Chlorine is a great disinfectant but hardens arteries, destroys proteins in the body, irritates skin and sinus conditions, and aggravates asthma, allergies, and respiratory problems. These are the same problems I've been discussing. Chlorine and bromine byproducts increase free radicals, aging and mutating cells while turning cholesterol (LDL Pattern B, more specifically) into the toxic substance Ancel Keys claimed it was. [55] Unfortunately, chlorine absorbs through the skin too, so a hot tub or shower is the same as drinking eight glasses a day. Chlorine and similar chemicals kill all the organisms, but it's like taking antibiotics. It helps for a little bit but then has long-term effects. Overuse is the problem. Chlorine gas inhaled while you shower increases absorption far more than drinking water does.

Additional water pollutants vary by location. Where I live, sodium is almost at the maximum containment level (MCL), presumably because we're almost surrounded by the Gulf of Mexico. Copper, radium, and fluoride are above levels I'd want to drink, and our area has also tested positive for E. coli and coliform bacteria, especially after rainstorms. My water company also pointed out that prescription meds increased 12% over a four-year period to 3.7 billion, so it's safe to assume that pharmaceutical waste in our water will continue to be a growing problem. [52]

I could continue for a few more paragraphs and discuss consumer product waste, organic solvents, and all the other lovely substances in our tap water, but that's not the purpose of this chapter. Nor is my goal to cast blame on EPA and the government or evil corporations. Nothing has the potential to derail natural health like picking a political framework to support it, just like not destroying the Earth became a discussion on party lines about carbon dioxide and climate change.

Bottled Water

We've all seen that kitchen sink water filter commercial where they talk about how many times you could circle the earth will all the plastic water bottles we consume in a year. It's unreal. As mentioned earlier, most bottled water is simply tap water with better PR and maybe some extra filtering. Not only are plastic water bottles dangerous for the environment, but one thing I learned from Daniel Vitalis is that water is a solvent. It's literally dissolving the plastic into your water or flavored drink.

Plastic water bottles increase your contact with petroleum based toxins. DHEP and other phthalates make plastic flexible, but cause cancer and reproductive problems. Phthalates are also common in beauty products. Lead, mercury, cadmium, arsenic, pesticides and herbicides can also leach into even bottled water and cause long term effects that are difficult to trace. [56] Although it's not the only substance that dissolves into our water from plastic polymers, the worst may be Bisphenol A (BPA), which disrupts the endocrine system to cause widespread hormonal problems systemically and at a molecular level. Water absorbs more BPA when plastics are heated. Because BPA targets estrogen receptors, even trace amounts can accelerate puberty in females and reduce differences between the sexes in body and temperament. It can also cause weight gain, but that's the least of the problems in my opinion. Younger children can't excrete BPA as well, but when Japan banned it in children's products, BPA levels decreased in people of all ages. Here in the US, 92% of us test positive for it because BPA is also in dental work, canned goods, toys, cell phones, and many other substances containing plastic. [57]

Keep in mind, BPA is just one of many potentially estrogenic compounds that can leach from plastic. Researching the number inside the little recycle symbol on your plastic bottles will let you know more about specific risks, but I find it easier to just avoid plastic bottles when possible instead of searching for bottles with "5", since the mythical "7" may or may not contain BPA.

We can't talk about bottled water without discussing flavored water or various vitamin waters. It's a lucrative gig—add a cent's worth of random, difficult to absorb chemicals to plain water and double the price. Drink companies are cashing in on this profitable industry, and their main goal isn't to properly hydrate you. This goes along with reading food labels and checking the ingredients. Don't be fooled by fancy phrases on the front of water bottle labels—check the ingredients to notice that colors and artificial flavors rule in the vitamin water world. I mean, what'd they do, drop a cartoon chewable vitamin in the water bottle and shake it up? Like I said earlier though, blaming companies or the government distracts us from personal choices that minimize toxic exposure.

I try to avoid plastic water bottles by reusing a small glass or stainless steel water container. When I'm at the airport I let them scan my empty glass water bottle during the security line then fill it up when the stewardess comes by in the airplane with the drink cart. Keep your heads up thirsty friends, there is a solution coming, I promise.

Which Water is Right for You?

Well Water

Let's start with well water. The advantage is no fluoride and you control the amount of chlorine. My husband grew up on well water and city water tasted like a swimming pool to him. The EPA recommends well water to be tested once a year because of the very real threat of contamination. Having a well reminds you that the actions of those around you can directly affect your health just like second-hand smoking. Like rain water, contaminants such as fertilizer and pesticides can end up in our water supply. It's tempting—everyone else in our neighborhood has lush, green lawns, and ours looks like a Chia pet with the mange. Well water can be beneficial or harmful depending on your area and your dedication to keeping the water supply clean. [42] Get your water tested to determine how it racks up, as the fertilizer a neighbor is using can seep into your water supply.

Spring Water

One of my favorite water choices is true spring water. After preparing my weapons of choice, I went on a water hunt, dragging my husband 40 miles south to a secret spring water location. Well, not that secret; there were a dozen people with five-gallon bottles lining up as we arrived. I did feel silly for going to all this trouble to procure the same amount of water the toilet flushed away every day. The feeling was similar to the sheepishness I endured a few months earlier sneaking around suburban neighborhoods to get my share of raw milk. After we filled 15 gallons worth, my husband took a swig.

"Tastes like water," he pronounced. I had much higher hopes for the curative properties of this particular batch of hydrogen and oxygen atoms, but soon realized that the extra minerals in the water from this particular spring had a slight laxative effect. Oops... Luckily, there were other water hunts that produced the best water we had ever tasted. It was hydrating and, dare I say it, alive. True spring water is not dug up like well water. This water is stored in giant aquifers miles below the earth's surface and is the other half of the condensation story you learned in fourth grade biology.

The Earth's Filter

I recently listened to Daniel Vitalis explain the complexities of spring water. Water is burned (oxidized) hydrogen. 90% of the known universe is hydrogen, as is 70% of the sun. In contrast, 60% of the earth is oxygen. Water is the ashes of hydrogen and covers 70% of the Earth's surface. The other side of condensation is infiltration. Water infiltrates the ground and journeys for centuries to form aquifers deep below the earth's surface. Even if polluted, water hits the ground and is treated by soil microbes, fungi, roots, sand, clay, and carbon deposits until it reaches an aquifer where it rests for thousands of years. Think of aquifers as giant underground bubbles filled with water. Water coming up from a natural spring after all those years in those giant aquifers is restructured, cleansed, and easily absorbed by your cells because of its perfect crystalline structure. It's as close as we can come to living water here on Earth. That screw on sink filter doesn't seem so sophisticated any more, does it?

Polluted water does not have the same crystalline structure. Crystals store information. Think of the delicate and organized structure of snowflakes or magnified ice. This is a similar concept to that of homeopathy—storing memories in water just like that pinpoint impression game. You know, the one where you make a fist and the pins make a 3D impression of it once you remove your hand. Our bodies are designed to drink pure, crystalline water. That's why most people groups built settlements around springs. Spring water is wild water.

Filters

Filtering is a start, but no two- or four-inch filter can do what the Earth can. Water is the Earth's blood and she does a good job of cleansing it. If you decide to filter your tap water, consider the water quality in your area first; this information is readily available via the internet, and every year you should get a brochure in

> Otherwise, we become like everyone else, shrugging off a $5,000 insurance copay but balking at the price of organic eggs.

the mail about your water quality. Also consider the economic costs and which filters you'll be able to install by yourself. Despite my common quip "Can you afford cancer?" to those grumbling about the cost of living healthy, we don't want to ignore the price of meaningful, lifelong changes. Otherwise, we become like everyone else, shrugging off a $5,000 insurance copay but balking at the price of organic eggs. Let's start by looking into alkaline filters, followed by carbon and reverse osmosis systems.

Alkaline Water

Alkaline water is currently the trendiest of all filters, the one with skinny jeans Instagramming filtered pictures of local art. At a basic level it makes a lot of sense; acid is bad and rising rates of kidney disease may be due to our acid producing diets. Making energy creates acid. Acid affects the body's delicate balance of protein creation and destruction. It is a byproduct of digesting proteins and most other chemical reactions our body undergoes. [48] However, the lungs, kidneys, and blood are excellent at maintaining a neutral pH of 7.4. Obsessing over whether every food is alkaline or acidic is asinine. It sounds like common sense, and it may be relevant in the lab, but in living, breathing humans it's much more complex than that. Likewise, pH values in isolation don't tell the whole story.

Conversely, our gut is excellent at temporarily sustaining us on a diet of fast food and soda, but soon something has to give. Although it's not a cure-all by any means, alkaline water is completely safe to drink. Again, researching whether each bite of food turns acidic or alkaline as different organs metabolize it takes the body balance conversation too far. Alkaline water is a high-quality option similar to reverse osmosis. They both filter water adequately but may need minerals added.

There are a number of filters that will adjust the pH of your water, talk to you, and do everything but clean the kitchen sink, since that's where they need to be positioned to work properly. Most of these filters are also capable of creating acidic water to accelerate skin and wound healing. Alkaline filters usually incorporate reverse osmosis or, more commonly, carbon filtration. There are some multi-level marketing systems (second only to politics as the bane of natural health) taking advantages of this latest fad, but an easier solution than cheapening alternative medicine wisdom with marketing tactics is to add a half teaspoon of baking soda to one gallon of water.

Carbon Filtration and Reverse Osmosis

I'll describe the process of carbon filtration and reverse osmosis separately because they work differently. The research I'm using is based on dialysis machines, which obviously need much cleaner water than what you drink every day, and also soften or deionize water to remove excess calcium, magnesium, and other minerals.

Carbon (actually activated charcoal) removes chloramine, one of those toxic chlorine byproducts, bacteria and their toxins, and other organic substances from the water. Carbon is very porous and has a high affinity for organic material, but can be contaminated with bacteria if not replaced as directed. These filters contain a separate filter to make sure your water doesn't taste like the crunchy center of a number-two pencil. Screw-on filters for your kitchen faucet are a stepping stone, like "water Febreze." They're not taking out all the fluoride, chlorine, or trace pharmaceuticals.

Reverse osmosis (RO) filtering uses high pressure to remove dissolved contaminants. Reverse osmosis wastes more water (three gallons to make one gallon) than carbon filtering, but the process eliminates many more toxins than department store filters you screw on the sink or attach to a water jug. RO filters push water through a membrane that stops any substance not named oxygen or hydrogen. Heavy metals ubiquitous in our environment are a subtle but dangerous health concern, and RO water can be part of the solution. The process allows aluminum and similar particles to be filtered out before they can cause anemia, bone weakness, and neurological problems. [53] RO filters filter everything out. Great, right? Unfortunately, this means you won't be getting any trace minerals from your water, and RO water may make you feel thirsty rather than hydrated. [54] Have patience. Common sense solutions are coming.

Practical Solutions for Your House

Whole-house, carbon-based filtering systems are readily available, but obviously this is an expensive way to make sure that even your toilet water is chlorine- and fluoride-free. Hardware stores now sell RO systems you can install under your kitchen sink. Many grocery stores dispense reverse osmosis water by the gallon. However, screw-on carbon filters specific for the tubs and showers used most frequently in your house are inexpensive, especially considering all the money you'll save on skin care. Many of them state they'll only last six months, and you should be able to tell when it's time to get new ones.

As you can see there are many different options for drinking water. You can harvest spring water or use alkaline or reverse osmosis filters. No matter which option you choose, I recommend adding minerals back into the water with one fourth teaspoon of Celtic, pink Himalayan, or Real Salt per gallon of water. You can also get Concentrace drops to add back in much needed minerals. Minerals make drinking water more hydrating.

I do need to add some caveats before you all rush out and drink a spring full of water. Just like a low-carb diet won't work for everyone, some of you will need to drink less than you are right now. Your water intake is closely related to the concentration of electrolytes in your body, hence the success of Gatorade and similar sugar water products. When it comes to water and how much water to drink there could be no greater controversy. You would think something as simple and available as water would be much easier to dose, but we are bombarded with a message that defies logic. We are told to drink water all day long regardless of our weight or how much salt we consume.

Are You Thirsty?

It's time to rethink how much water you are drinking. Have you been counseled to drink at least eight glasses of water per day? Or maybe you were told to take your body weight in half and drink that in ounces per day. I have a problem with that amount of fluid entering your body and so does your metabolism. But wait, isn't drinking plenty of water throughout the day good for our metabolism? People who are at a healthy weight didn't get there because they drank tons of water throughout the day. As controversial as this may seem, downing quarts of water does not flush fat out of your body or increase metabolism. [59] The cutting-edge science responsible for eight glasses a day is from 1945! If you only drink plain water you aren't actually hydrating your body or your cells, you are simply peeing it out and taking some important electrolytes with it. In fact, I just heard a story about a baseball player who died because he only drank water on a hot day and didn't replenish his electrolytes.

Extracellular Fluid

Water just doesn't go into one compartment once ingested. We have about 15 liters worth outside and in between our cells. This is called extracellular fluid and it includes our blood. Our cells maintain the balance of fluid inside and outside of cells using sodium and potassium. That's why prescribed IV fluids containing a salt solution when we're hospitalized. If they just poured water into your bloodstream, the change in electrolyte concentration would force so much water into your cells that they would burst like a water balloon. So much for avoiding sodium, huh? I get some seriously weird looks when I tell some clients we are going to increase their salt and decrease their water consumption. This recommendation is not for everybody and we'll get more into that.

One key point I want you to gather from this book and use when reading any health information is simple yet powerful. Stop and think about how that information applies to you and your health. Maybe someone else needs to hear it but you've already applied it earlier in your journey. If your drink of choice is soda or alcohol then it will need to be swapped out for water, but someone who has been resisting salt, has hypothyroidism, or is cold all the time needs to rethink proper hydration.

Overhydration is a Real Problem

This would be a good time to talk about overhydration. I see this among my most motivated clients who have wholeheartedly listened to dietary dogma for most of their lives. Most of us have heard that we are already dehydrated if we only drink when we are thirsty. So are you telling me we shouldn't eat when we are hungry but before? It doesn't make sense, and it's not backed by science either. [60] Similar to hunger cues, the body tells us cues when to drink and, if we are paying attention, when to stop.

We are all aware of how we feel when we overeat and we know the consequences of too many calories. It's a bit different when we drink too much water. Besides metabolism and activity levels, it involves your heart, skin, kidneys, and the absorptive capabilities of your intestines. Part of my husband's job is to give patients the specific fluids and electrolytes they need during surgery. He says that when a patient is given an IV solution, much of the extra water only stays in the bloodstream for a few minutes before taking the path of least resistance elsewhere.

If the patient is face-down for surgery, excess fluid quickly swells the soft tissues of the face until they look like the Michelin Man. Over-hydration leads to congestive heart failure, heart rhythm disturbances, poor wound healing, and other issues that sometimes require complex interventions. Relatively healthy people are not going to get swollen ankles from drinking one cup of water too many, but the principles remain. Our food provides plenty of water too, so as long as you drink more than the 500 milliliters we urinate every day, the body can regulate itself just fine. [61] In fact, I have some of my clients monitor their urine color to make sure it stays yellow.

Don't Pass the Salt Substitute.

My grandparents have used one of the most expensive seasonings in the world. Both of them have landed in the hospital for low sodium levels because years ago they heard eating too much salt was bad for them. Healthy sodium levels should be anywhere from 134-145. At the time we dashed my grandma to the hospital after acting confused and blacking out, her level was 125. She drastically reduced her salt intake for years and drank water religiously throughout the day. Grandma's doctors swiftly told her Gatorade would be the best beverage of choice. The commercially available electrolyte drinks are simply flat sodas with extra food coloring. Of course, I got to work making her a homemade version with salt and lemon juice which you can find in the recipe section. But how would I know that my fragile grandmother needed less water and more electrolytes? Ultimately, you need to know when to become more concentrated or more dilute at any given time.

Sally Slurpee and Debby Drought

There are two types of people in this world: those who need to drink more water and those who require electrolyte water with salt added. Just like exercise, our culture thinks that more is always better. If you're like my client Sally Slurpee—that's her real name, I swear—

coffee, orange juice, and a tall glass of water are all emptied before work every morning. Lunchtime comes with iced tea and free refills, and before bed we also had to account for two glasses of wine, two bottles of water, two additional glasses of water, and a mug of hot tea.

Sally resembles the awkward commercials for bladder medicine because she has to search out restrooms wherever she goes. The burden on her kidneys flushing her system so many times a day is only matched by her serious electrolyte deficiencies, which has slowed down her metabolism and obliterated the ability to listen to her body's needs. I didn't let Sally drink anything but the rehydration drink, and only four ounces at a time. I taught her mindfulness and being in the moment, asking herself, "Am I thirsty and do I need to drink this?" instead of reflexively downing liquids.

If your urine is clear and a two-hour car trip involves bathroom breaks, it's time to slow down on the beverages. Other signs to note if you are overly hydrated are cold hands and feet and a temperature always below 98 degrees. For many clients, vegetable juicing has been a life saver to truly hydrate their systems. If you are one of my close friends or family members, you've probably received a juicer or smoothie maker from me for Christmas or your birthday at some point. However, not everyone tries to drink their way to health. If you have to force liquids past your lips, perhaps you resemble Debby Drought.

Debby only drinks half a cup of black coffee for breakfast, a can of diet soda at lunch, and one glass of wine at dinner. Like Sally, Debby Drought has an electrolyte imbalance, but the problems here are completely different. Debby doesn't feel cold all the time, but she gets dizzy and has frequent headaches. Her urine is dark and she's not drinking enough hydrating fluids. I told Debby to consciously notice if she feels thirsty, monitor her urine for a healthy yellow color, and start substituting better choices throughout the day. Since Debby doesn't like to drink fluids, we started slowly by incorporating more soups and bone broths before adding in spring water and some rehydration drink recipes she could enjoy.

Eventually, both Sally and Debby were able to drink and enjoy plain filtered water at some of their meals. As their electrolytes balanced, they learned how to regulate their fluid intake more naturally. Just like counting calories is difficult to maintain, concentrating on your water intake only works long term if your body learns to sense your fluid and electrolyte balance. That's why I haven't urged you to restrict your fluids or drink a glass of water when you wake up every morning. Listen to your body throughout this entire process. None of us should take this journey to wellness alone. Bring that concept to the subject of filtering your water or changing the source. Talk to your family and come up with the solution that works best for all of you. There's no need to slam this book shut and run to the hardware store to pick out the best whole-house filtration system they sell. With water, ease your way into health, but start today.

Action Step: Mindful drinking

- Conduct an ice cube tray experiment Dr. Emoto would be proud of and see for yourself if water changes because of a label. Label each cube in the tray with a different word such as love, forgiveness, peace, hate, or sadness. Fill the tray with water and let it freeze. You may never feel the same about water again! Who knew water was so sensitive?

Action Step: Curious if there's a spring near you?

- Go to findaspring.com and find out. You can also buy raw water, but hunting it yourself is much more fun and economical.

CHAPTER SIX

Real Exercise

Not a Fan of Exercise Either?

"Before my treatment plan with Melanie I could not run or jog without nausea. I was an avid runner and became depressed. My monthly cycle gave me out of control mood swings, horrible cramps that left me crying myself to sleep at night, and bed bound for 1-2 days with pain. I also could not eat without having reflux which also disturbed my sleep. I can now exercise without throwing up or having an upset stomach afterward and I can eat food without discomfort. My period is regulating—I only ever felt this way in the past on birth control pills! I'm so happy my money is being well spent on actually healing my body than the years I tolerated hearing I was over reacting or needed multiple medicines." Guerda Merilian

Exercising has not always been a favorite pastime of mine. I wasn't the athletic one growing up unless you count a short stint in cheerleading and baton or summer camp activities. I would get really excited about a new running plan and quit after a month's worth of boring jogs. Or I would get super attached to one piece of workout equipment at the local gym for three weeks and then never return. I always had these high hopes of continuing all my adventurous workout routines, but never seemed to stick with them for more than a few months. I never spent enough time to really see the results that I wanted. The core issue was a true dislike of exercising. I practically cringe just saying the word "exercise"—it brings to mind pictures of long, grueling cardio sessions that made me feel utterly exhausted. Today, I often say instead that I'm committed to movement as a means of health promotion. I recommend that everybody incorporate some kind of physical activity into their daily routine. Besides keeping you lean and fit, exercise has so many other health benefits and that is what this chapter is all about.

The statistics are surprising since research clearly shows that physical activity improves physical and psychological health and well-being. Studies in North America and Europe confirm that 85% of adults don't get the recommended amount of exercise and only 40% have any interest or intention to exercise at all. [62]

There's a reason why the food and nutrition chapter came before the exercise chapter. We've all heard people say, "I can eat or drink whatever I want today and I'll run it off tomorrow," or "I'll do an extra fifteen minutes of cardio so I can eat that cake." Unfortunately, it doesn't really work that way. In order for our bodies to be healthy and perform optimally, it all starts on the inside. "But, wait a minute," I can hear you saying, "Isn't this chapter about exercising?" Yes, it is, but I want to make sure you're aware that you can't work out enough to make up for a bad diet. Healthy diets first, then exercise second.

Movement: Make Time to Live.

Did you know that even walking a few times a week has been shown to increase our lifespan? [63] When my husband and I were in Greece, we walked everywhere. Even when we caught the subway it was a 20-minute brisk walk. I felt amazing on that trip partly due to our healthy diet, but also because of all the walking we did. We didn't notice many overweight people either, and I believe it is because of all the walking they do. Exercise doesn't have to be something where you schedule in 45 minutes of cardio or weight training. Sprinkle movement into your day several times a week and before long it all becomes a habit and a lifestyle.

> *"For 3 years I had arthritis so bad that it looked and felt like my hands were broken. All of my doctors said, "You have rheumatoid arthritis. Take ibuprofen." My ability to hold my children, care for my family, and do simple mundane tasks like getting dressed was also progressively getting worse and spreading. This was NO way to live! Now I have complete range of movement in my hands, and I have been pain free! Although Melanie has added much to our lives these last few years in the way of relief, encouragement, prayers, information, dedication, and especially patience/unending creativity when working with our children, the greatest thing has been Hope. Hope that we would feel better and hope that with hard work we would be able to live a more normal life. Praise be to God for struggles, for hope, for relief, and for people like Melanie that shine light in dark places!"*
> *Amy Bodkin*

It isn't hard to eat well or create time to get fit. Deeply engrained in our culture is the concept, "If someone really wants to do something, nothing is going to stop them." Well, when you become aware of how much health and fitness enhances all aspects of your life, you will want to do it, and you will create the opportunities to eat well and exercise. We all know exercise can help us lose or maintain a healthy weight and prevent osteoarthritis and heart disease, but knowing those facts won't get us off the couch. So what will?

Culture Lies.

Looks can be deceiving. Our culture has an unrealistic drive to be thin, and thin doesn't necessarily mean healthy. Getting skinny should never be the only goal when choosing to add more movement into our lives. I've had slender female clients and muscular male clients suffering from cancer, hormone imbalances, and severe infections. Health is not about the number on the bathroom scale or a defined six pack.

Instead of a quick, overnight change, our goal is holistic weight loss—a gradual and steady process of making our bodies wholly stronger. For many people, their symptom of imbalance is gaining weight, but that doesn't make them necessarily less healthy than the person with indigestion or a weakened immune system. Your goal shouldn't just be to lose five pounds; working out should be utilized as an anti-aging and longevity tool. When we perceive working out from a holistic mindset, movement has the added side effect of improving our appearance. Being skinny can mask our health problems just like pharmaceuticals can. We have to lose the prejudice in our society that smaller people are healthy and can eat junk food simply because they are thin.

High-Stress Aerobic Exercise Isn't Worth It.

Here's a secret: going from 90% organic, nutritious, real food to 100% isn't really going to unleash a new level of perfect health. Even more so, going from regular movement and exercise to marathons and endurance races isn't going to exponentially make you that much healthier. The goal is to work with your body. In nutrition, sometimes people get carried away with a concept and end up not helping themselves. With exercise, it's the idea of whipping yourself into shape. I know people who were sick and felt that working out would pump the sickness out of them. It is possible to stress the adrenals with vigorous workouts and cause an imbalanced endocrine system. [64, 65]

That's not to say I'm against exercises based on high intensity. In fact, high-intensity workouts are great for short periods of time with plenty of rest in between. Use functional movements that work holistically rather than set patterns on only a few muscles. Functional exercise movements like **CrossFit** have really started a revolution for the "rest of us" without expensive equipment or much experience. However, it is time to focus on being balanced in exercise too. Choose a workout that is forgiving on your body. Exercise isn't an end to itself; it's another piece of the puzzle of longevity, wellness, and even beauty that comes naturally when incorporating these principles. On the opposite side of the spectrum, sedentary lifestyles can be just as dangerous as over extending ourselves. Sit at home and watch TV eating kale chips all day and you'll starve yourself spiritually and emotionally as well. A sedentary lifestyle coupled with healthy eating means you're still missing out.

For an example, my friend Dr. Tom Schneider describes how he lost over 100 pounds after he started doing triathlons and quit smoking and drinking. Sounds great, right? The truth is he actually got sicker because he never dealt with his imbalanced lifestyle of punishing his body with stress and a brutal work schedule. [66] Overdoing it with exercise before taking care of leaky gut or hormone imbalances will cause even more damage. Another possible reason for people getting sicker from extended periods of maximal exercise is faulty studies. We've been looking at cholesterol levels instead of weakened immune systems and increased inflammation. As mentioned previously, low cholesterol isn't proven to lower the incidence of heart disease and heart attacks. We Americans just love isolated numbers that are supposed to represent our health status. It is better to check **homocysteine levels** and **oxidative stress**. Hear me out; we do need to incorporate exercise into our lives, but high-stress aerobic exercise doesn't seem to be the best option for many people. Of course, if the goal is to lose weight while still eating the Standard American Diet, anything short of strenuous exercise multiple times a week rarely changes the numbers on the scale.

Hormones Matter.

Hormones play an important role in exercise. The human body loves homeostasis so much that it often sabotages attempts to burn fat and get healthier. Insulin, leptin, glycogen, and other proteins do a remarkable job, but the complex interplay between the gut, nervous system, and endocrine organs such as the pancreas and thyroid is vulnerable. Once again, the secret is to work with your body, making sure that the autonomic nervous system knows when to burn energy and when to relax, when to store energy and when to freely release it. While strenuous physical activity can be a great form of medicine, many people have so much stress on their body—social, spiritual, and physical—that attacking health problems with intense exercise makes things worse.

The impact of overtraining extends to multiple hormone symptoms. When I test hormone levels, the majority of my clients who exercise frequently exhibit high cortisol, suppressed testosterone, and low **DHEA** (which converts to estrogen, progesterone, and testosterone). As you exercise, testosterone increases as it repairs the body and builds stronger muscles. Continued overexertion stresses the body and slows testosterone secretion, stopping the repair. The last thing we want is heightened catabolic activity (breaking down large molecules into smaller ones to release energy) without an off switch. Comparing levels of testosterone and the damaging stress hormone cortisol show if it's time to put down the weights and hang up the running shoes for a few days. Overtraining increases the risk of injuries and a multitude of health problems as testosterone levels plummet and cortisol levels rise. [67] It seems counterintuitive to recommend that someone wanting to lose weight should *rest* and substitute softball or hiking for high-intensity cardio. And speaking of rest, sleep comes first when balancing hormones, as we'll see in the therapy chapter.

> Your social networks may matter more than your genetic networks. But if your friends have healthy habits you are more likely to as well. So get healthy friends. – Mark Hyman, MD

I'm not saying exercising is bad, but if you are not seeing expected results, it might be time to limit the frequency or duration of your high-octane activities and get your hormones checked. Albert Einstein once said that the definition of insanity is doing the same thing over and over again while expecting a different result. It may be time to try something new.

Time & Motivation:
What Was It You Were Waiting for Again?

Many people will tell you, "I know I need to work out, but I just don't have time." I want to ask them, "Do you have time to be sick? Do you have time to have a shortened life?" When it comes to living a lifestyle of movement, it requires commitment and the ability to prioritize. We somehow have time to spend hours on Facebook, but not for a 15-minute stretching routine? We have to realize that we do have time. The journey to wellness is much easier if we take the time to enjoy it. We were created to live, move, work, and play, not sit around going from computer to phone to tablet.

Living an active lifestyle does not mean you have to be a gym rat and work out an hour every day. In fact, I propose much less for clients who are starting from a lifestyle where the only exercise happens if the remote control runs out of batteries. Especially for them, too much exercise can put unnecessary stress on the body. Movement in our lives should be as routine as brushing our teeth. The solution is the same as altering food habits. To change your diet, do one thing and master it, such as following my bone broth recipe at the back of the book. Before long, you're making bone broth every week in the crock pot. Exercise is exactly like that. Start with one small goal such as, "I'm going to walk 10 minutes today." You can do that. Put it on the calendar that you will walk 10 minutes every other day this week. It's that easy.

The other aspect that we must face in order to begin working out is motivation. Maybe before even thinking about what type of exercise you would like to start, ask yourself, "Why should I work out in the first place?" Science shows that telling people to watch for more subtle benefits of exercise increases the likelihood they will stick with it, even without the immediate weight loss they might otherwise expect. Being in tune with our body gives us important feedback about the effects of these new habits. Coupled with the expectation of outcomes is self-efficacy. This is the perception that any person can accomplish exercise and is why they should start with "movement" instead of exercise. [68] For example, my assistant at The Grecian Garden is a yoga teacher named Meagan. She'll start her students with really simple postures to build their confidence and poise before stretching them (literally) into more elaborate and contorted shapes. You have to walk before you can climb walls or CrossFit your body into shape.

None of us like being told what to do. Viewing exercise as a "have-to" activity and an excruciating means to an end decreases your chance of sticking with it. That's what makes natural health so hard for some people. Rather than a "take this pill and don't worry about it" mentality, most of what I'm suggesting in this book requires subtle yet ongoing activities. In fact, significant research points out that doing what someone tells you instead of internalizing and individualizing your workouts is one reason gym dropout rates are so high. A solution is to find intrinsic motivation, which means finding a way to exercise that's enjoyable and sustainable without placing external pressures, such as society's fickle demands, on your fitness routine. That's why I'm encouraging you to get healthy and stay healthy through exercise rather than appealing to your extrinsic need for tighter abs, shapelier quadriceps, and similar concrete reasons to embrace fitness. Those easily defined goals are more motivating in the short term, but two years later very few people with that sort of reasoning still exercised regularly. [62] When you make it your own, you are much more likely to easily incorporate it as a continual habit.

> Two-thirds of those with arthritis, lupus, fibromyalgia, and similar conditions are obese, but less than half of those 45 million Americans have been educated about the increased abilities that regular movement and weight loss can provide. [69]

Starting from the Bottom

I've geared this chapter for those of you who don't exercise consistently, but I want to briefly explain the benefits to the sickest and most senior among us.

My husband wrote a medical article about preventing older people from falls and injury, and he was surprised at the pivotal role of exercise and diet (I wasn't.). Regular exercise decreases other risk factors for falling, including cognitive decline, osteoporosis and chronic disease. Exercise prevents or slows disability and can restore function so patients can once again perform activities of daily living like dressing themselves. The key is to find movements that those across the health spectrum can perform. For those in long-term care facilities, walking, tai chi, and especially individual programs targeting areas of concern such as gait or range of motion decreased injuries the most. In the community, programs that incorporate more than one type of exercise have better results in lowering fall risk and number of falls, but any fall prevention program that includes regular movement can expect a reduction in fall risk by a fourth, especially if balance and gait exercises are included. [70]

> "The power of healing is within you. All you need to do is give your body what it needs and remove what is poisoning it. You can restore your own health by what you do—not by the pills you take, but by how you choose to live." —Terry Wahls, The Wahls Protocol: How I Beat Progressive MS Using Paleo Principles and Functional Medicine

Nine Reasons to Stay Active

1. Reduces Stress

It's no surprise that most Americans are stressed out; in fact, eight out of ten of us are. That's pretty much everyone. Leading a high-stress life has been dubbed the silent killer. Exercise doesn't just help your body: your mind benefits as well. Have you ever been stuck thinking about a problem over and over again and decided to go on a walk? After the walk your mind was calmer and the problem seemed to solve itself. I mentioned in previous chapters we do live in a toxic world. Toxins such as those from heavy metals or pollution put extra stress on our bodies. One of the easiest and most effective ways to rid our bodies of toxins is to sweat. Sweat the toxins and stress away. Exercise at the appropriate duration and intensity for your fitness level (and how well you're eating and sleeping) reduces and normalizes cortisol levels. This makes it easier to lose weight, relax, and handle all of life's changes.

2. Improves Sleep

De-stressing through exercise also improves sleep, although heavy exercise just before bed may make it difficult to fall asleep. Allow time to wind down and relax. Though exercise is a key factor, the body also uses diverse clues, from colors and the amount of darkness to hormone levels, to discern when it's time to sleep or awaken. Even the most natural sleep aid can become a crutch, so try to paint a stark contrast between active and resting phases. It's going to be hard to convince your body it's time to sleep if you've been studying or watching movies in your bed all day. Exercise is especially important if your schedule requires you to travel often or work night shifts. Rather than spending a mindless half hour on a treadmill, research shows that brain-stimulating exercise such as exploring or climbing improves sleep and protects us from age-related cognitive decline. Exercise benefits for the aging brain depend on the accompanying cognitive load. [71] Simply put, mind and muscle use equals restorative sleep.

3. Tones Your Body Inside and Out

You already know by now that true health comes from the inside, and that nutrition is key to being healthy. The added benefit of exercising is toning from the outside in. While your muscles on the outside are being toned by weight bearing exercise or Pilates, your internal organs are getting a workout and massage too. Yoga massages all the internal organs and glands of the body thoroughly and in a balanced way. Remember, you can eat the healthiest food on the planet, but if your body isn't digesting and assimilating it, what benefit are you having? Certain sequences in yoga actually help to improve blood flow to the digestive tract and other organs. Even the muscles inside your blood vessels learn to relax. [72] When you incorporate an active stretching routine you will soon notice improved flexibility, increased mobility, a calmer mind, and a de-stressed and relaxed body. However, the reasons behind our enhanced levels of health are less understood. Most of us simply feel better; our digestion improves, we are less prone to illness, we have more energy, and our bodies seem to function more efficiently.

4. Sustains Energy

Living an active lifestyle which incorporates movement is the best way to sustain energy. Without some form of exercise, we can create a vicious cycle by covering up our low energy with coffee and sugar which stress the adrenal glands, recreating the problem every day. It's not normal, despite the advertisements, to need little bottles or huge cans of energy drinks to get you through the afternoon. We were not created to have such drastic dips and surges of energy throughout the day—pay attention to the affect your diet has on your energy as well. If your diet is nourishing, but you still have fluctuating energy levels or trouble sleeping, work with a holistic practitioner on slowly incorporating physical fitness as your hormone levels improve.

Exercising to get more energy only works to a certain point, however. Good gut flora smooth out energy levels as well. Although exercise is a very important part of a healthy lifestyle, I've worked with clients who are personal trainers and athletes, but still have fluctuating energy levels. I attribute this to over working their bodies to the point that stress and other hormones become imbalanced.

5. Releases Emotional Freedom

Our emotions affect us at such a deeper level than we often realize. Some emotions are in the forefront of our mind while others are more subconscious and behind the scenes. In either case, exercise is a positive release to help balance our emotional life. It doesn't require you to work yourself to death to get this emotional cleansing from exercise; research shows that the intensity of exercise doesn't relate to the undeniable emotional benefit it provides. In one study, participants who ran slowly received the same emotional benefit as those who ran at a faster pace. [73] We're going to go much deeper in a subsequent chapter about other tools to help with emotional release. However, the interaction of emotions and activity only grows stronger the stronger your physical body becomes. I interviewed professional soccer player, fitness model, and counselor Junior DeSouza for one of *The Nourishing Podcasts*. He mentioned how he's had to pause his sports career at different stages to deal with emotions before they sabotaged his performance or wreaked destruction on other areas of his life. Think of all the tragic mistakes athletes have made because they failed to understand that the physical body, emotions, and the spiritual self are all connected. My co-host on The Nourishing Podcast, Emily Morgan, is healthier now that she understands these truths than she ever was playing soccer.

6. Improves Oxygenation

Take the deepest breath you can. Let it out. Didn't that feel good? Dr. Weill recommends you substitute oxygen for that cup of coffee to help you focus. We are oxygen depleted. Deep breathing expands the lungs, decreasing your risk for pneumonia just like moving water prevents algae from growing on the surface. Oxygen kills germs (and fat too), but wait a minute before you run off to an oxygen bar or steal Aunt Mabel's oxygen canister! All the benefits from oxygen are available from the plain 21% available in every breath you take.

Breathing releases toxins because your lungs are an elimination organ, just like your liver and kidneys. My husband carefully adjusts his patients' breathing parameters during surgery so they inhale and exhale the right amount of oxygen, carbon dioxide, and anesthetic gas. Unlike the kidneys and blood, the lungs can adjust our acid-base balance very rapidly. Carbon dioxide is an acid and a waste product, regardless of your opinion on climate change.

7. Controls Appetite and Weight

Exercise regulates key hormones leptin and **ghrelin** (That's not a typo, though it'd be more fun if they were called gremlins.). Although exercise may seem to make you hungrier, this isn't necessarily true. Incorporating more movement makes it easier to consume fewer calories. You may notice when you work out that you actually end up craving more nutrient-dense foods. The best way I can explain this is when I work out I don't want a McDonald's cheeseburger afterwards. What I want is an avocado-topped salmon burger with steamed broccoli on the side topped with butter and a large spoonful of kimchee.

Have you ever seen runners finish a race and then see who could drink the most beer or suddenly down a pizza post-race "because they can?" Working out is one of the most beneficial elements to create a healthy environment in your body. Don't ruin the moment. Listen to your body and don't be afraid to ask yourself as many times a day as necessary, "What am I hungry for?" Your body will tell you. Dig under those initial cravings for a Snickers bar or a bag of Cheetos to find what your body is truly saying. Do you need more protein? More fat? Fat is the most satisfying component to any meal, so don't be afraid to add extra coconut oil, avocados, or butter to your meals, which can keep you from snacking more.

8. Regulates Insulin Sensitivity

Exercise improves insulin sensitivity through glucose transport molecules in the individual cells of your muscles. Cells use glucose for energy instead of letting it sit in the blood stream. Excess glucose in the bloodstream is harmful long term, which is why insulin encourages cells to take and use it. Think of a school bus that stops at every kid's house instead of releasing a whole swarm of them at the bus stop. Each "kid" arrives at home where they belong. The end result is useful, available energy instead of fat storage. Movement also affects your full range of hormones positively relating to accessing stored energy and regulating how the energy is used. This is critical for someone wanting to lose weight. For example, I've seen tremendous progress in my practice with women who have been diagnosed with Polycystic Ovarian Syndrome (PCOS) by taking a holistic approach and also balancing their blood sugar. One way we did that was by incorporating yoga into their fitness routine. A study comparing yoga to regular exercise in teens with PCOS found that insulin resistance, glucose, and lipid levels all decreased in those doing yoga. [74]

9. Improves Bone Health and Body Composition

We've all heard that weight bearing exercise is excellent for long-term bone health, but what you may not know is that exercise (or the lack thereof) is in fact a bigger determinant of osteoporosis risk than diet. Your hormones determine the shape of your body and your hormone balance or imbalance is determined by diet and lifestyle among a few other contributing factors. Keeping your hormones balanced will give you the body shape that you want much easier than some fashionable exercise that singles out a particular muscle group.

Find Out What Works for You.

There are so many different forms of exercise—I always look at the business cards pinned to the bulletin board at the local health food store when I forget that. You can go to a local gym for a class, swim laps at the community rec center, or simply go for a hike. I love walking. Whatever you choose, be consistent in your efforts to move. As mentioned earlier, motivation comes when you find lasting reasons for why you want to work out. I'm not going to explain all sorts of different exercises in depth, but a few deserve an honorable mention. Ultimately, it's up to you which movement you incorporate into your lifestyle and I hope I've inspired you to do so.

Before you pick up those weights don't forget about an important first step. Another reason aches and pains are associated with exercise is improper preparation. Don't avoid exercise for weeks yet dash off and play three hours of soccer without stretching beforehand. A proper cool down period after exercise is paramount for strenuous activity. I get strange looks at the grocery store because of the large amount of Epsom salts I buy at one time, but your muscles crave magnesium after exercise. The body quickly eats through fat and nutrients during a workout, so replenishment is key.

Yoga

Yoga is something that I wish I'd started sooner. Growing up in a Christian home though, yoga was not welcomed. In a small Amish town near where I grew up, the only attraction besides a cheese factory in the area was a simple bookstore, and that's where I found the book *Holy Yoga* by Brooke Boon. She claims that yoga movements are just another way to praise God with our bodies. I was skeptical at first, but soon discovered that my back pain disappeared, my muscles strengthened, and I was breathing deeper. I routinely suggest yoga to clients, and for those skittish about that kind of environment, I recommend Holy Yoga.

Many believe that yoga is rooted in Hinduism, but Hinduism's religious structure actually evolved much later and incorporated some of the physical practices of yoga. Traditional Yoga is the discipline of unifying the body, mind, and spirit. As Brooke Boone states, "In Holy Yoga we pursue unity of body, mind, and His Holy Spirit that dwells within us, with the intent of worshiping and serving Christ with our entire being." [75]

Yoga can be practiced by anyone at any age. I've done yoga stretches with my infant nephew and have clients in their seventies practicing it. Yoga is built on three main structures: physical postures, breathing, and meditation. The postures (or poses) in yoga are designed to put pressure on the glandular systems of the body, resulting in more effective total health. During yoga, muscles are stretched and contracted, creating space in the joints which increases elasticity and range of motion. Another aspect of yoga is the breathing techniques used. These are based on the concept that breath is the source of life in the body. The two systems of poses and breathing prepare the body and mind for meditation. Some meditate on nature, specific words, or even Scripture. I choose to meditate on God's promises. Consistent everyday use of yoga can produce a calm clear mind and a strong capable body.

Yoga therapy has been developed to address many health challenges including chronic back pain, asthma, depression, arthritis, high blood pressure, digestive disorders, etc. Yoga not only has benefits for our physical body but there are mental and emotional benefits as well. It removes stress, calming the body and mind while simultaneously strengthening core muscle groups. Virtually everyone who does yoga for a period of time reports a positive effect on their personal outlook. Regular yoga practice can create mental clarity, relieve chronic stress patterns, relax the mind, and sharpen concentration.

Martial Arts

I interviewed a local sensei about karate and taekwondo. Studying the martial arts is a phenomenal way to exercise if your diet and hormones are in balance. Isometric exercises, long periods in demanding stances and plenty of calisthenics improve flexibility and strength. For a less combative approach, tai chi involves a series of movements performed in a focused, deliberate manner. I was intrigued because it seemed slow and meditative but really strengthens your core. Tai chi developed as a way to disguise martial arts techniques while still promoting strength developed from a mind-body-spirit connection. It's relaxing, calming, reduces stress, and is simple enough for use by elderly patients to decrease their fall risk. [68]

As many of these **Eastern** modalities are holistic and incorporate emotional and spiritual components, you'll want to read the section of this book devoted to spirituality and remaining true to your beliefs.

Pilates

Growing up, my siblings and I used to watch and laugh at infomercials. You know the ones I'm talking about (Edible hair removal from Australia, anyone?). Anyway, I had seen the infomercial for Windsor Pilates and knew I needed to try it. For Christmas that year, I unwrapped the Windsor Pilates VHS collection and couldn't believe how simple yet challenging the movements were. Pilates definitely strengthens the abdominal and other core muscle groups and uses breath (a key element) along with the stretches for improved posture, toned muscles, and a flatter tummy—all while not leaving the comfort of a mat.

If yoga is not something you are comfortable with, try Pilates. It can be done by all fitness levels. German athlete Joseph Pilates created a series of mat exercises designed to help balance the body, improve motion, strengthen and promote mental and physical harmony. Initially, dancers chose Pilates for its concentrated movements, deep stretching, and focused breathing. But soon word caught on that it wasn't just for dancers anymore. Pilates requires proper alignment and breathing, which make it a great choice for a small, instructor-led class or one-on-one training. [76] Even my husband can follow along with the movements, and he professes to have the kinesthetic learning abilities of a tree stump.

T-Tapp

"Tuck tuck tuck, tuck those buns. Knees out, knees out, keep those knees out!" You will have that phrase stuck in your head for days after doing T-Tapp.

This is one of my all-time faves. At first, I thought it was a little cheesy with its aerobics class feel that seemed to appeal mainly to women. Then, I found out more about T-Tapp from Dave Asprey, "The Bullet Proof Executive." He says it's one **biohack** of an exercise and that you really can do less while achieving impressive results. T-Tapp is a totally different type of work out. T-Tapp can help you lose weight, strengthen your spinal alignment, and has the added benefit of lymphatic pumping to help detoxify. Creator Theresa Tapp wanted to create something accessible by people of all body shapes regardless of their starting fitness level. The goal is to lose inches rather than pounds as the exercises gently trade fluffy fat for dense muscle. T-Tapp can help you lose weight, strengthen your spinal alignment, and has the added benefit of lymphatic pumping to help detoxify.

Lymph moves when you do, and proper circulation and drainage of the lymphatic system is crucial because your brain uses the lymph system for immunity as well. The blood brain barrier prevents all but a select few substances from entering the brain but this newly discovered lymph pathway into the brain and spinal cord proves how connected even the most isolated organs are to the rest of the body. [77] All of a sudden, it doesn't seem so ludicrous that mental illness improves after dealing with an underlying infection or that depression and anxiety vanish after simple supplementation.

No matter which type of movement you decide to incorporate into your life, I want to stress the fact that exercise doesn't have to be spending an hour at the gym three times a week or doing intensive cardio routines every day. When it comes to working out, doing small amounts of high-intensity exercise is plenty given that your diet is healthy and that you are getting adequate rest. Some of you may be in a different place and need to work with an expert for your specific needs, but whatever you choose find something sustainable and something that you love.

Here in the Florida Panhandle, I tend to see clients at opposite ends of the exercise continuum: they only exercise if chased by a bear or alligator, or they exercise continually and hope it'll make up for a poor diet and other health issues. I do offer both groups hope though. I'm not telling anyone they have to give up the strenuous workouts that they love permanently. However, it's time for all of us to start back with the basics, making sure we have the nutrients we need to foster healthy endocrine and hormone systems so our body doesn't tear themselves down in the process of forming killer abs or defined triceps.

**Action Step: Write out your motivation
and set your motion goals.**

This is one step to write out because without the reason why, your goals will likely not be met. So what is your motivation to begin incorporating movement in your life? Maybe you've noticed tight muscles or joints upon standing or maybe you're trying to balance your blood sugar. Know what is motivating you and what kind of exercise you would most enjoy. The next step is to set up an achievable goal. Write out in your planner or weekly calendar a form of movement you know you can accomplish such as walking around the neighborhood with your significant other or doing a short workout video Monday, Wednesday, and Friday.

Action Step: Get a workout partner.

- Start thinking of friends or family members who would be fun to work out with. We get lazy without accountability, and studies show that those with workout partners exercise much more consistently.

CHAPTER SEVEN

Real Medicine

After seeing Melanie for my thyroid I went to my doctor for a checkup and some lab testing. He told me my thyroid and other results were all "perfect" but that he noticed I hadn't filled a prescription in 3 years. He said, "Whatever you're doing, keep doing it". Melanie found a candida infection and a wheat sensitivity. She has me taking a few herbs and supplements, but more importantly she has helped me change my diet. Melanie showed me that food really can be my medicine. I can feel the difference and my physician approves. Thanks Melanie!" Sally Mason

"What seems toxic to one organism may not seem so to another. Can you drink red wine without getting a headache? How much coffee would it take to give you the jitters—half a cup, or maybe you can drink it all day? Each individual's personal detoxification response is tied to genetics, lifestyle, and diet." - Dr. Jeffrey Bland MD

You've made some dietary changes, hunted for spring water, and did your first T-Tapp workout, but you still have a cold. This is where natural medicine comes into play. When you get sick, start coughing or sneezing, or suffer digestive upset from spoiled food, what's the easiest solution? Isn't it quicker to run to your very own natural medicine cabinet rather than trying to make an appointment to see your physician while you still have symptoms? You'll most likely hear one of three things: "It's viral. There's nothing we can do. Drink more fluids and rest." Or secondly, "Here are some antibiotics." Or finally, "Here are antibiotics and anti-inflammatories." All three of those prescriptions combined won't help your body become stronger after the initial episode is over. Taking too many antibiotics (Haven't we all?) can lead to drug-resistant bacteria, allergies, decreased immunity, and skin reactions such as eczema and digestive problems. Yes, you heard me right, all of the above can happen with the overuse of antibiotics. Friends, there is a time to take antibiotics and it is rare.

There are so many other things we can do to help our body when we come down with something. Try the garlic tea featured in the herb section of this chapter, pick up some elderberry syrup for your child's cough, or see below for my favorite probiotics. It's time to take medicine that will help us without harmful tradeoffs. The goal in natural medicine is prevention and we already learned a large piece of the puzzle is diet. A nutrient-dense, toxin-free diet avoids foods that tend to weaken the immune system, such as sugar, unprepared grains, industrial seed oils, and processed and refined foods.

Why shouldn't we just keep taking pharmaceuticals like candy? Most medicine your doctor prescribes used to come from a natural source but is now synthetic. For example, a whole class of medications, local anesthetics, originated from the numbing properties of coca leaf extracts.

> Thankfully, since then science has produced agents safer than cocaine to numb the body.

Thankfully, since then science has produced agents safer than cocaine to numb the body. We need medicine and science. Rather than clashing with natural therapies, the two can work together with an integrative approach. Using both worlds, we can get to the root of a problem quickly which will naturally take care of symptoms as opposed to simply chasing them. Not everything traditional cultures passed down as medicine is legitimate and accurate. We are better educated today than ever. The information at our fingertips is astonishing to think about. Science backs up natural options as well; one of my favorite websites to prove this is https://naturalmedicines.therapeuticresearch.com/.

Whether we intend to or not, many of us in natural health use an integrative approach. I often recommend blood or saliva hormone testing to a client right after I muscle test them. I truly believe we need both sides of the coin. We need the mainstream medical field for emergencies such as broken bones, and we need functional medicine doctors to review our lab work.

Natural medicine allows us to take our health and put it in our hands. We are responsible for our health, and while holistic practitioners can help us on the journey, **it really comes down to how we live our lives day in and day out.** The

> Stocking your alternative medicine cabinet is about empowering you to take control of your health via safe, natural methods.

best way to utilize this next section is not to go to the store and buy everything listed. As you become more educated, the next time a headache or a stomachache returns, choose one of the options below instead of popping another antacid or ibuprofen. Remember, you know yourself and your sensitivities best. All of this is not intended as medical advice and the methods I plan to highlight are not necessarily the same individual items I would recommend if you came to see me. Stocking your alternative medicine cabinet is about empowering you to take control of your health via safe, natural methods. This chapter could technically be several books in itself, but for each section I'll only give a brief introduction and further reading if necessary.

How Is Herbal Medicine Used?

My office is located in an herb store. Everyone who walks in says, "It smells so nice in here! What are you making?" The always helpful owners of Old Thyme Remedies, Theresa and Beth, usually smile and say it's simply the blended fragrance of all the herbs they sell. The feeling of working in a place with that much happy plant material always brightens my mood. It truly is a magical place.

Most of us are familiar with taking herbal teas such as peppermint when we have an upset stomach, but herbs can be used for so much more. I can remember making my nephew dill seed tea to calm his upset tummy when he was just a few months old. Herbs are a powerful group of medicines that can be used safely and effectively. If you are adding oregano and basil to your spaghetti sauce or drinking a cup of herbal tea each afternoon, natural medicine is already a small part of your life and you may not have even realized it. Conventional medicine is very effective at handling life threatening situations or broken bones. But what about a cut, or scrape or a runny nose? When I was younger we always reached for the antibiotic ointment or over-the-counter antihistamines. Over time, those medicines (chemicals) are simply stopping the symptom without promoting actual healing.

Learning to use natural medicine is like learning to ride a bike for the first time. After all, there are probably more tinctures, oils, and herbal capsules lining Whole Food's shelves than there are illnesses in the world! Well, maybe not, but it can definitely be overwhelming. When I first started learning about herbal medicine and wild herbs I thought," Why didn't I grow up learning this?" These secrets were lost with our grandparents and further back. My grandmother tells me stories about her grandfather picking wild herbs and making them teas when they were sick. At this point, you may need to decide which products are truly medicine and which are mostly tubes of petroleum wasting space. Of course, you'll want to toss out expired meds, but I'm thinking that ibuprofen, antacids, and cold medicines need to be used a lot less often.

God created the Earth in all its beauty, with stunning sunsets and picture perfect landscapes, and if we look closer, there's medicine everywhere. It's time we all went through a relearning process on what true medicine is. As always, this information is intended for educational purposes only and I recommend further reading at the end of the book if you want to research a specific topic.

Essential Oils

These are top picks for my medicine cabinet. I used essential oils for the first time when my natural doctor recommended I make a blend of thyme, oregano, and cinnamon in a carrier oil and apply it to my feet and stomach every night. Essential oil application far exceeds home remedies. In fact, two breakthrough medicines for leukemia are derived from the traditional healing properties of rosy periwinkle essential oil. [78] These drugs work synergistically with other natural products, demonstrating that plant-based therapies have complex uses far beyond home remedies and minor health problems. [79] Essential oils truly are in a class all their own. Through the process of distillation they can be made from seeds, bark, stems, roots, flowers, and other parts of plants.

From emotional healing and mood elevation to skin concerns and infections, essential oils are great to have at a moment's notice for the following reasons:

- They are a unique concentrated medicine, which is why oils work so effectively in our bodies. This is also why I don't recommend using them internally. Inhaling, **diffusing**, or applying topically are the best routes of administration.
- Essential oils have the ability to cross the blood-brain barrier and promote natural healing in many key areas of the brain due to their teeny tiny molecular size. This has been a game-changer for those with autism and ADHD.
- As plants with certain genetic characteristics flourish, their oils can continually mutate and morph to stay ahead of "superbugs." Oils have been proven over and over to kill viruses and bacteria, while synthetic medicine is the same formula each and every time and does not have the ability to adjust if a virus decides to mutate.
- Other than skin irritation from certain undiluted oils, there are few possible side effects.

Safety

I like using oils every day for prevention, and when an illness arises. There are books and so many resources on essential oils today that I would need to write a sequel to give the subject justice. Some of the highest-quality oils aren't always the most well-known, however. Beware of marketing ploys when it comes to essential oils. Besides inflating prices, most of these companies advocate internal use of essential oils, which I do not think is safe without the supervision of a qualified healthcare practitioner. It takes 16 pounds of peppermint to make one ounce of oil! [80] I find applying oils topically, inhaling, or diffusing them is much safer and more effective. My favorite place to apply oils is on the bottoms of the feet, where the largest pores in our bodies exist. Recently my husband came down with a nasty stomach bug. I quickly gave him some viral immune stimulator homeopathic and then covered his feet and chest in essential oils. Immediately, he said he felt better and believed the essential oils were a big part of that. There is no denying their efficacy, and you don't need someone selling you oils to tell you that. To further study essential oils I recommend the book *The Complete Book of Essential Oils and Aromatherapy* by Valeria Ann Worwood. Below are some of my favorite oils and how I use them.

Peppermint: Tummy, Headaches, Nausea, Dizziness

Three of my top uses for peppermint essential oil are for headaches, nausea, and dizziness. Do you have a tummy ache? Peppermint to the rescue! Be careful though because peppermint is strong and irritates sensitive skin. Most adults are fine applying it neat (undiluted) on the temples or stomach, but children or more sensitive individuals and need it diluted in a bit of olive oil.

Lavender: Soothing, Sleeping, Bath

So calming, this essential oil is great for a relaxing bath or insomnia. The anxiety-reducing properties of lavender aren't just psychological: it even relaxes smooth muscles of the heart and blood vessels. [81] Inhaling this soothing floral scent can calm you down after a rough day. Add a few drops to a bath or even to your pillow for a quick rewind. Have you ever held a baby and knew they were moments away from sleep? We used to waft this scent towards my niece and nephew's tiny noses to help them rest.

Eucalyptus: Chest Rub, Coughs, Spiders

Dealing with a chest cold or sinus infection? Eucalyptus diluted in olive oil rubbed on the chest or inhaled can quickly alleviate upper respiratory complaints. My go to use for eucalyptus is to keep spiders and other bugs at bay while I'm earthing. I love going outside and laying or sitting on the ground barefoot. Apply a few drops of eucalyptus to the towel that you bring outside with you—it will keep bugs at bay, both the ones you can see and the microscopic ones you can't. [82]

Tea Tree: Disinfectant, Anti-Fungal

Ahh, the smell of clean! This is a wonder disinfectant and I've used it to clean my entire home. It smells fresh and light but it can be a powerhouse when it comes to cleaning. I add a few drops to a sink full of hot water and go to town scrubbing. I swear I can hear germs fleeing when I use it. Tea tree oil can also be applied to fungal infection on the skin or feet, although I do not recommend applying tea tree near the face as it can cause burning. Use caution with this one when applying topically as a dilution in olive oil may be better. [82]

Rosemary: Headaches, Alertness, Sinus

Trouble focusing? Know someone with ADD or ADHD? Give them some rosemary essential oil to smell. It's great at helping kids focus on their schoolwork and completing tasks. A friend of mine has her son wear a pewter necklace that has a spot to put essential oils. She uses rosemary or vetiver to help keep her son focused. Rosemary is also great to use for a headache. Apply to temples or diffuse while resting. Sinus headache relief from a Neti pot gets even better with a drop of rosemary.

Frankincense: All-Around Amazing

This is my first and the best choice with which to start building your essential oil collection. I've used it on my face neat for a sinus headache. I rub this one on the bottoms of my feet regularly, and I love frankincense during a yoga session or when praying. There's such a spiritual quality about this one that's hard to describe. It must have been special since it was a baby gift for Jesus. Frankincense is extracted from the boswellia tree and is excellent for pain and inflammation. [83]

Homeopathic Remedies

History of Homeopathy

The roots of homeopathy stretch back to the days of my probable great Uncle Hippocrates, who theorized a healing method by "similar." Later in the seventeenth century, the father of homeopathy Samuel Hahnemann proposed the first law of homeopathy as "like cures like." The standard medical assumption had always been that if the body produced a symptom, it was the opposite medicine to that symptom that would cure it. For example, constipation would be treated with laxatives. Hahnemann called his system of healing "homeopathy", from the Greek *homoios* (similar) and *pathos* (suffering or disease). [84]

> "To carry this truth further, we have found in natural medicine, what heals the disease also prevents it."

"To carry this truth further, we have found in natural medicine, what heals the disease also prevents it." Hahnemann's methods were ridiculed by his colleagues, but patients flowed in and the results were astonishing, further bolstering his theories. By 1892, homeopaths controlled 110 hospitals, 145 pharmacies, and numerous orphanages, nursing homes, and insane asylums. Hahnemann prescribed one remedy at a time, while conventional apothecaries made fortunes by mixing numerous substances and selling multiple potions for each ailment. Hahnemann believed that symptoms were much more than just annoyances to be suppressed—they served as clues on how the body wanted to fight off the underlying problems. The apothecaries were giving noxious substances and often new symptoms would appear. Hahnemann and his followers successfully treated cholera, yellow fever, and scarlet fever at rates far beyond their contemporaries. [85] If you want to dig deeper into using homeopathy for your family, I highly recommend *The Complete Homeopathy Handbook* by Miranda Castro.

Diluted but Powerful

Homeopathy can be successfully used for coughs, runny noses, bruises, the flu, food poisoning, etc., but the right remedy must be chosen. Homeopathy takes into consideration personality traits and other symptoms present when figuring out which remedy is best. You may have seen some allergy medicine at the health food store and it said "homeopathic" on it, which means that an herb, mineral, or animal tissue is diluted to the point where that original material can no longer be detected. This is a great stumbling block for any conventionally trained scientific mind. They will wonder how something so diluted could possibly work. It seems more often with the case of homeopathy that if you haven't experienced its healing in your body you really don't believe it. There is though a pharmacological law that helps us understand how this works. If a large dose of poison can destroy life, and a moderate dose will paralyze, then a very small amount will actually stimulate those same life processes. Some theories even suggest that the dilution process triggers imprinting which directly affects the electromagnetic field of the body. In any case, homeopathy can work safely and effectively. This effectiveness does not mean that a homeopathic should be compared to prescription medicines, because they do work differently.

Potency

All homeopathics are made similarly—e.g. belladonna steeped in alcohol for a period of time before it is strained. This starting liquid is called a tincture. Then 1/10 of the tincture is added to 9/10 of alcohol and shaken vigorously (succussed). This first dilution is called 1X. The number of a homeopathic remedy reflects the number of times it has been diluted and succussed. [86] For example, Arnica 6X has been diluted and succussed six times. There is also a centesimal scale (one part tincture in a hundred) as well as an M scale (diluted a thousand times). These high potencies also have a greater dilution, which by homeopathic philosophy makes them stronger than tinctures that are less diluted. Extreme dilution enhances the medicine's healing properties and eliminates undesirable side effects. The most common scale used is the decimal scale with 6X, 12X, and 30X being the most common. M (a thousand times) and CM (100,000 times) dilutions should only be used by homeopaths and not the home prescriber.

Constitution

One other point I want to make about homeopathy is that is takes into consideration the whole person. This means your constitution and other symptoms can all be a factor in choosing the right remedy. I really enjoy this aspect of homeopathy. More often than not people have a doctor for every part of their body, but looking at the body holistically and realizing everything is all connected can mean a solution can be found much sooner. In homeopathy we look past the presenting complaint or disease and try to find a remedy that matches the totality of the symptoms. In this regard, there are usually many more questions to ask to determine the best remedy. [16]

The Law of Cure

The law of cure is based on Constantine Hering's detailed clinical finding about curing sick patients. As someone is cured, symptoms move from the innermost organs of the body (those most vital to life) to the outermost. In other words, cure moves from "within" to "without." Cure takes place from above to below so that symptoms start clearing from the head and work their way down to the feet. Symptoms that have been suppressed in the past often resurface during the process of a cure and usually do so in the reverse order from their original sequence. Hypothetically, if a patient with heart disease had been successfully treated with orthodox medicine for a stomach ulcer before the heart condition, then the appearance of a stomach symptoms (less severe than the original complaint) would be a welcome sign that the old suppressed symptoms were being cleared out.

> Symptoms that have been suppressed in the past often resurface during the process of a cure and usually do so in the reverse order from their original sequence.

The suppression of a disease usually leads to further complications. The law of cure echoes the homeopathic principle that diluted substances, even pharmaceuticals, influence the body's healing response. [86] You don't have to choose homeopathy to fix the problem, and you can live a healthy life and never take a homeopathic remedy, but when you have symptoms homeopathy is a great place to start. I always keep homeopathics in my natural medicine cabinet. They are safe to use and even sensitive individuals can benefit from them.

Choosing Homeopathics

Okay, now that we are a little more familiar with homeopathics and how they work, it's time to stock some of my favorites into your medicine cabinet. Homeopathics can come in little pellets or in the form of a liquid alcohol base. The remedies below are made by Professional Complementary Health Formulas. I test my clients for homeopathics and the ones below seem to work almost universally. I also stock the ones below in my personal medicine cabinet and find that this really covers a lot of bases. You can find similar formulas at health food stores or by contacting Professional Complimentary Health Formulas to find a practitioner in your area. All of Professional Formulas' homeopathics are alcohol-based, which means they are lactose free and dosing instructions are listed on the bottle. For kids who cannot tolerate the alcohol being held in their mouth or under their tongue you can apply it directly to their skin.

Airborne Allersode

One of my favorite blends used for those suffering from seasonal or indoor allergies. Doesn't it make sense to decrease your sensitivity to these items as opposed to taking a drug that only stops the symptoms? This one helps to decrease sensitivity to common inhalant or airborne allergens from trees, flowers, grass, weeds, dusts, molds, and animals. This remedy has helped many cat allergy sufferers!

Biting Insect Mix

A client of mine has a beehive and got a sting that swelled her entire hand and wrist. She took the biting insect mix drops and the swelling disappeared. These drops help to decrease your sensitivity to many different types of insect bites and are especially helpful for people who get large welts from mosquito bites.

Bacterial Immune Stimulator

This is one remedy to always have on hand and is a godsend for anyone suffering with a bacterial infection. My pregnant sister took this remedy once she found out she tested positive for Strep B. At the time of the birth, no Strep B was detected, which prevented her son from needing antibiotics after birth. This remedy also comes in handy with babies as it can be applied directly to their skin if a bacterial infection is present.

Bowel Pathogen Nosode Drops

Most people have all manner of parasites, bacteria, and viruses invading their gut. When these bad bacteria get out of hand, reach for bowel pathogen nosode. It increases immunity to common bowel pathogens.

Food Poisoning Detox Drops

Enough said. You know after experiencing one bout of food poisoning you wouldn't wish it on your worst enemy. So the next time you think you've been poisoned or ate bad food, start with these drops.

Food Additive Detox Drops

These are a lifesaver for the sensitive individual trying to remove food additives, preservatives, and colors from their diet because they have a reaction when they eat the smallest amount. These are especially helpful after eating out. You've chosen the cleanest thing on the menu, but you know you're reacting to something that was one the plate. These drops will help aid in the detoxification and relief from food additive sensitivities including sulfites.

Rescue Remedy
(Not Made By Professional Complementary Health Formulas)

This flower-based remedy was created by Dr. Bach to deal with emergencies and crisis. It can be used to help us get through any stressful situations, from last-minute exam or interview nerves, to the aftermath of an accident or bad news. Rescue Remedy helps us relax, get focused and get the needed calmness. It comes in spray, drops, cream, or in pastilles. There are many other Bach flower remedies—check out bachflower.com to learn more.

Cell Salts

The "Homeopathic" system of the Cell Salt remedies was developed by Dr. Schuessler, a German doctor in the late 1880s. He analyzed the ash residue of human cells and found 12 inorganic mineral salts. He theorized that these 12 elements are critical to balancing cellular activity and health and made 12 homeopathic remedies with low potency to be assimilated rapidly and easily. They have shown to be helpful in balancing many conditions in the body. The strong point of using the cell salts is building up a person's constitutional health over a period of time. Homeopathy raises individuals' vital force while the cell salts help to rebuild. In a way the cell salts are the "vitamins and minerals" of homeopathy. You can take a Cell Salt remedy for six months to a year for supporting a chronic problem. For example Calc Fluor and Calc Phos are excellent to help the teeth and bones. Serum Phos is great for inflammation and anemia. You can choose the individual cell salt remedy based upon your symptoms or you can choose the cell salt combination formula that has all the remedies. A great place to find out which cell salt is best for you is schuessler-cell-salts.com.

Herbal Medicine (Tea, Tincture, Syrups, Flowers, Herbs, Etc.)

A common criticism of herb safety is that supplements aren't regulated by the FDA and that potency and quality differs drastically depending on variables such as the part of the plant used and how it was grown. These fears are unfounded if you select the companies I mention in the resources at the end of this book.

Herbal medicine is much older than Hippocrates, but continues to increase in popularity. It is affordable and increasingly accessible. There are three main ways you can begin incorporating herbs into your everyday. First, you can plant an herb garden. Second, wild foraging is becoming increasingly popular especially with the help of herbalist taught classes. Third, purchasing herbs is easy to do through trusted sources.

Selecting medicinal herbs to include in a garden is easier than you think. Basil, mint, horseradish, and other common plants have practical, curative, and, more importantly, preventive uses. Despite my company's name, I'm not an expert at bringing plants to life, so the ones that do survive in my yard are resilient and tenacious. Wild plants have high amounts of antioxidants making them hardy and disease resistant. That same tenacity is passed on to us when we eat them. This doesn't mean that dill planted in the lawn will have superpowers if it survives the lawn mower.

I recently completed an edible gardening class that helped me understand how to grow plants in my area. A local nursery can explain specific soil and climate needs. Raised beds or simple designs may work best to grow easy herbs such as sage, lavender, or peppermint. [87] Certain herbs flourish in the shade, while others enjoy hot climates. For extra points, upload pictures of your herbs to social media so everyone can see how health-conscious you are—just kidding.

I get so excited when I see wild dewberries turn from red to a deep purple color. After picking, I give them a quick rinse and culture them to make probiotic-rich smoothies and pancake toppings. Wild foraging can be a fun way to connect with nature. Attend a local herb walk to familiarize yourself with which plants are edible and which plants aren't safe to consume.

If gardening or wild foraging doesn't sound like an afternoon of fun you can always purchase herbs through your local herb shop or online through Mountain Rose Herbs. Local herb shop, health food stores, and co-ops are invaluable because they usually offer classes and workshops on how to make and use herbal medicine. I like to think of herbal medicine as a gift from God. The Earth is literally covered in plant-based medicine! Below are some ways to easily incorporate just a few herbs into your natural medicine cabinet.

Elderberry Syrup

Elderberry, where have you been all my life? This is possibly my most used herbal remedy! Elder flowers are a wonder for colds, flu, upper respiratory infections and fevers. Elder has immune-enhancing properties and you can make a very potent, safe and effective tea or syrup. Elderberries support and increase immune function and contain antibacterial and antiviral properties. I have an elderberry syrup recipe in the recipe section of the appendix. If you're not up for making your own, simply pick up a bottle of elderberry syrup at your local health food store.

Arnica

As a topical cream or oil, spread arnica on muscle pain, bruises, or any type of trauma. I've found that it greatly reduces healing time or bruises and sore muscles when applied right after injury. You can either use a topical cream or take homeopathic pellets to take internally. The pellets are great to take before and after surgery or dental work.

Calendula Salve or Tea

Great for healing the skin and promoting cellular repair, calendula is antiseptic and commonly used externally for bruises, burns, sores, skin ulcers, eczema, and psoriasis. Calendula can be applied topically in either salve or oil form. It is also used internally for gastrointestinal issues and is wonderful for healing the stomach lining. It can be taken in a tea for fevers, cramps, indigestion, diarrhea and leaky gut. It also promotes lymphatic movement.

Stinging Nettle Leaf

This herb is a mineral powerhouse high in iron, calcium, potassium, silicon, magnesium, manganese, zinc, and chromium along with a host of other essential nutrients. It increases metabolic activity and strengthens and tones the entire system. It is useful for growing pains in young children, achy joints and arthritis, reproductive health, and alleviating PMS and menopause symptoms. It is also indicated for liver problems or congestion and to treat allergies and hay fever. Nettle has antihistamine properties so it can work great for itchy skin. It's effective as a tea, tincture, in capsule form, or even made into a syrup or **glycerite** for kids.

A great combo to help with seasonal allergies is one that contains nettle, **quercitin**, and bromelain (the enzyme found in pineapple fruit). This type of supplement can be taken preventatively or when symptoms start. Avoid quercetin during pregnancy.

Garlic Tea, Oil

Garlic should be your best friend and if you take it in high doses, it may be your only friend. It kills all the bad germs while supporting beneficial bacteria. You're probably already using it to season your food but I personally believe we can never have too much garlic. Try making my garlic lemon tea (located with the recipes in the appendix) at the first sign of a cold or for overall immunity.

Garlic oil is the go-to remedy for earaches. A few drops of oil are put into the affected ear (as long as there is nothing draining from the ear canal and the ear drum is intact). Garlic oil can be purchased at the health food store and usually contains mullein, tea tree, or other infection fighters.

Oregano Oil Pearls

Are you seeing a trend? A lot of these are for the immune system and oregano oil is no exception. There's a reason we Greeks are healthy and immortal; well, we have high life expectancies, anyway. Greeks drink a mountain tea that contains wild oregano. Taking oregano pearls are the safest due to the capsule preventing any irritation. Oregano is a great addition to any anti-microbial protocol.

Mullein

Mullein is an unsung hero in the herbal world. It can be applied topically to bug bites to help pull out toxins or it can simply be boiled for a throat-coating cough syrup.

Ginger

Tea from fresh ginger alleviates nausea, colds, fever, indigestion, and menstrual cramps. Ginger supplement capsules relieve headaches and achy joints, and even ginger candy can relieve motion sickness.

Chamomile

Also a favorite among Greeks, a sweet calming cup of chamomile tea can solve so many problems from tummy aches to trouble falling asleep. It's a must have and it tastes good.

Astragalus/Echinacea

The immune-boosting king and queen! I'm including both of these in the same section because they both take down coughs, colds, and the flu. Teas, tinctures, and capsules all effectively support immunity.

Peppermint

My favorite use of peppermint is as an essential oil. Of course the tea is excellent too. I find the essential oil applied topically works much quicker. I've also seen peppermint work effectively for dizziness caused from a virus or from spinning in circles on my office chair. Not me, silly! My nephew!

Licorice Tincture, Tea, Capsule

Licorice is an adaptogenic herb which means it can help our bodies' response to stress. The extract can be used for extremely low cortisol. The DGL (deglycerized) form is a safe and natural alternative for heartburn and acid reflux. Licorice tea is also a very effective natural anti-inflammatory that soothes sore throats and coughs. Avoid licorice if you have high blood pressure.

Slippery Elm

Slippery elm lozenges are great for a cough or sore throat. Slippery elm made into a tea is great for digestion as its soothing for the entire digestive tract. It has been used for reflux, ulcers, diarrhea, and constipation. It can be taken as a lozenge, tea, or tincture.

Cramp Bark, Jamaican Dogwood, Black Cohosh

I combined all of these herbs because as tinctures either taken combined or individually they work great for pain from menstrual cramps, headaches, body aches, or muscle pain. You can take 20-60 drops of the tincture of any of these or a combination four to six times a day. Avoid taking with sedative medications. [88]

Honey

It's the perfect addition to your afternoon tea or the best way to sweeten your lavender lemonade. Honey can also stop a middle of the night cough in its tracks. But seriously, this stuff is liquid gold and no kitchen or medicine cabinet should be without. Local wildflower honey is effectively used for seasonal allergies but I learned so much more than that from my local beekeeper during his recent class.

Propolis has proven antibiotic and antiseptic properties and may also have antiviral and anti-inflammatory effects. It makes the hive stronger because it is derived from sticky sap from pine trees and forms important structures in the part the hive where bee babies are born in a germ-free environment. Bee babies just sound so cute and fuzzy! But I digress. Propolis does have quite a bitter taste, so once I bring it home from the grocery store, I cut it with raw honey on a spoon and say, "Open wide!"

Manuka honey doesn't play around. Manuka honey is great to have on hand for skin infections and has even been shown to kill staph infections. So slather it on and cover with saran wrap because it's going to be one long sticky night. Honey has long been used to treat chronic wounds, and more recent studies shows that both propolis and manuka honey provide immunity to viruses and bacteria commonly affecting the mouth and throat. [89]

Vitamins and Other Supplements

Stocking a natural medicine cabinet with essential oils, homeopathics, and herbs is a great start. Listed below are a few other important supplements with bioavailable recommendations. There are a few below that were so important they needed an honorable mention.

Vitamin C

Vitamin C is important for so much more than immunity. Vitamin C plays a key role in the health of our adrenals. When it comes to vitamin C whole-food sources such as camu berries, rose hips, or acerola powder are best. I like The Synergy Store brand Radiance C or Garden of Life Raw C for supplemental options. Take up to 1,000 milligrams of whole food Vitamin C daily for maintenance.

Minerals

I could write a whole book on minerals. Just like a car needs a key to work, so our bodies need minerals. Minerals are the key that make enzymes work and enzymes are essential for all chemical reactions in the body. To give another analogy, if our body is a brick house, minerals are the mortar that keeps it held together. Magnesium, iodine, and zinc deficiencies are quite common. Testing is key when it comes to minerals. A hair mineral analysis test is invaluable for knowing which minerals we should be supplementing with. Many are supplementing with too much calcium, which can cause hardening of the arteries and kidney stones. I included a chart at the bottom with food based sources of minerals which is usually a great start when it comes to restoring minerals. Often, we can become so depleted that supplements are necessary along with food sources.

Minerals are under looked but they are the unsung heroes of our health. A fascinating resource about misconceptions is the book *Calcium Lie* by Robert Thompson. As I mentioned in our conversation about seaweed, iodine can be a tricky mineral to supplement, so check out *The Iodine Crisis* by Lynne Farrow for more information.

What depletes magnesium?

- Pharmaceuticals
- Calcium, supplemental
- Vitamin D3, supplemental
- Copper, unbound
- Caffeine, nicotine†
- Dehydration, sweating
- Phosphates
- STRESS

Magnesium can be supplemented orally or topically, and some prefer topical applications to avoid having to take another pill. Magnesium CALM is a great drink sold at almost all health food stores that can be a relaxing way to end your day. There are several different forms of magnesium in supplement form and each has its own unique benefits. Magnesium taurate is a great magnesium supplement for additional heart support. Magnesium glycinate in capsule form is an excellent evening choice. My clients with fibromyalgia report less pain when taking yet another form of magnesium: malate. This version is energizing so take it in the morning. Magnesium is often absorbed better through the skin and there are several topically applied magnesium oils and lotions on the market that are easy for those not wanting to take another supplement.

One point to make regarding cramping legs is your cortisol levels. If cortisol is too high, potassium can be depleted, causing cramps. A trace mineral supplement with potassium comes in handy for those situations. The mineral zinc boosts the immune system tremendously. Along with other minerals, make sure its bioavailable; I recommend zinc picolinate. Finding a zinc with B vitamins, especially B6, increases the body's ability to absorb this needed mineral.

Nutrient	Sources	Nutrient	Sources
Trace minerals	seaweed, bone broth, stinging nettles, kale, parsley, unrefined sea salt; liquid minerals	**Zinc**	oysters, beef and lamb, zinc picolinate, ionic zinc
Vitamin B6	seaweed, bone broth, stinging nettles, kale, parsley, unrefined sea salt; liquid minerals	**Magnesium**	raw pumpkin seeds, dark chocolate, stabilized rice bran, seaweed, pine nuts
Boron	trace minerals, prunes, raisins, ionic boron	**Iodine**	sea weed, scallops, cod, yogurt; trace minerals, ionic iodine
Bicarbonate	baking soda	**Sulfur**	garlic, onions, cabbage, kale, eggs
Sodium/ chloride	unrefined salt	**Selenium**	Brazil nuts, blackstrap molasses; ionic selenium

Potassium	orange juice, coconut water, sweet potatoes, blackstrap molasses	Vitamin C	citrus fruits, peppers, kiwi, papaya, pineapple; whole-food vitamin C (created with low heat as heat above 105 degrees F damages vitamin C)
Calcium	dark, leafy greens, broccoli, dairy	Vitamin A and D	cod liver oil, high-vitamin butter oil, pastured butter, pastured animal lard, egg yolks

Probiotics

Our microbiome is fascinating. We have around one trillion bacteria living on our skin and in our gut. Due to excessive antibiotic and antibacterial use, these beneficial microbes largely responsible for balancing our immune systems have taken a hit. As I already mentioned, the best way to improve our beneficial bacteria is through probiotic rich foods so that these beneficial microbes have all the nutrients they need to survive and thrive in our gut. Cultured vegetables or kefir are excellent options when it comes to probiotic rich foods. Probiotic supplements can also assist in restoring our microbiome. I prefer professional formulas such as Prescript-Assist or the Klaire Labs product Ther-Biotic Complete. Prescript-Assist probiotics are soil-based and most of my clients do very well on them, regardless of digestive issues or even histamine sensitivities.

Enzymes

Everyone needs enzymes. I have never thought that there was one supplement that could benefit everyone, except for enzymes. Some people need stomach enzymes, others require small intestine enzymes, and for others, pancreatic enzymes are key. I test all my clients to see which ones they need. People often tell me that they've tried enzymes and they didn't work—the ones they took originally weren't the specific type they needed. [90]

Bentonite Clay

Who knew eating dirt could be so much fun? The miracle of bentonite clay goes back to electrons and positive and negative charges. Bentonite clay is negatively charged and toxins tend to have a positive charge. Bentonite clay is a swelling clay, much like a sponge. As it reacts to water, its pores absorb toxins from the body. Special kinds of clay and dirt act as a filter, taking

Bentonite clay can be effective regarding the following issues:
- Allergies
- Providing minerals for the body
- Speeding up recovery from vomiting and diarrhea
- Detoxification
- Oral health preparations
- External use for all types of skin problems and to speed up healing

out the bad stuff. It's been used as a healing agent for millennia, as the upcoming documentary *Eat White Dirt* will explain about the mineral kaolinite. We are seeing a resurgence in ancient medicine and clay is one of the oldest and most effective when it comes to purging the body of toxins. I realize this is the exact opposite approach to using antibacterial soap to clean off dirt. [91] Our sterilized society has yet to realize that the elimination of all microorganisms is not helping our immunity. It can be used for a fantastic detox bath, but I've also been called a "mud mouth" for using it in my homemade toothpaste.

Activated Charcoal

Activated charcoal may sound like an odd thing to have in the medicine cabinet. It can be used for bloating, upset stomach, or even food poisoning. For acute use, charcoal is useful in cases of intestinal illness, vomiting, diarrhea, and ingestion of toxins without respiratory complications. It is always a good idea to keep the local poison control number on hand in case a child ingests a toxic substance. Immediately take a child to the hospital if he or she has swallowed anything of concern rather than playing doctor at home. Obviously, I recommend that same approach to any sudden health problem that could rapidly worsen while you're waiting for natural medicine to gently take effect. Activated charcoal is something to have on hand when there is no time to get to the health food store. You will be relieved that this safe and natural product is in your medicine cabinet should the need arise. [92]

Cod Liver Oil/High-Vitamin Butter Oil

I know it was a long time ago, but remember what Dr. Price said? The fat-soluble activators vitamins A and D are where it's at. Okay, so he didn't say that verbatim, but he meant it. Recent science explains how crucial vitamin D is to boosting the immune system. It affects white blood cells down to a molecular level and signals them to gear up and kill foreign invaders. In the future, over and underactive immune systems could potentially be brought back to alignment with this knowledge. [93] Our fear of the sun has led to an epidemic (and I don't use that word lightly) of vitamin D deficiency. This is where high-quality cod liver oil can be very useful. I recommend traditionally prepared, fermented cod liver oil and while we're at it, let's mention the ever-loved sister to cod liver oil, high-vitamin butter oil. These two combine to pack a powerful punch.

Colloidal Silver (Liquid and Gel)

No, it won't turn you into a Smurf. Well, it could, but only if you ingested an amount high enough to give you heavy metal poisoning. In the case of colloidal silver, the silver content should be measured in parts per million and you need to get it from a reputable source, such as Sovereign Silver. Silver doesn't require much time to kill germs and reduce inflammation, so it's a novel way to eradicate infections without worrying about antibiotic resistance. [94]

Castor Oil Packs

This old fashioned remedy still deserves a space in your modern alternative medicine cabinet. Both Chinese medicine and **Ayurvedic** medicine support the use of castor oil packs because they promote healing and reduce inflammation. Castor oil packs can be done right before bed as they are relaxing and take self-care to a whole new level.

The packs are said to improve elimination and circulation, especially of the lymphatic system. Other ailments castor oil packs aid include liver disorders, pelvic pain, tendinitis, kidney stones, fibroids, ovarian cysts, swollen joints, and digestive disorders, but more studies are needed to validate all of these claims. [95]

The packs are created by placing castor oil-soaked flannel over your abdomen or affected area. Cover with a small sheet of plastic, and then an old towel. Place a hot water bottle or heating pad on top. Leave the pack on for 45-60 minutes. Read a book, write out some action steps, or catch up on your favorite Netflix. You'll want to wear an old shirt as castor oil can stain fabric.

Should We Completely Turn Our Back On Modern Medicine?

I personally do not condemn anyone for seeking practical and scientific help with their illness. God has given us life and that it is our duty to safeguard that life by whatever reasonable and wise course is open to us. I feel as though I've been entrusted with the gift of health and I'm not about to abuse it. For me, that means using natural remedies whenever possible and the thought of taking a prescrip-

"What we have now is doctors who are actually better technically at what they're doing in their specialty than 30 or 40 years ago, but we lost the relationship, when the doctor would look people in the eye and say, 'I care about you. We can do this together.'"—Dr. Oz

tion drug has not crossed my mind in years. But everyone is at a different place and that is okay too.

Remember, supplements can cover up symptoms if we are not careful. If problems persist after using a remedy, seek appropriate natural health care advice and possibly get a second opinion. Whether using home remedies or not, getting to the root problem is always ideal.

Action Step: Update your medicine cabinet.

- Go to your medicine cabinet and toss out all the expired meds. Replace with homeopathic and other natural remedies.

Notice what you tossed out. Were there pain relievers, itch creams, or sinus meds? Next time you're at the health food store, pick up a few homeopathic remedies in place of the ones you threw out. Dosing information is on the box and can be safely incorporate into your routine.

If you would like a visual of how to make tinctures and other herbal medicines, check out my video series on Natural Medicine and Health Products (http://www.ehow.com/video_12305740_herbal-preparation-medicinal-plants.html).

Chapter Eight

Therapy for Wellness

I've had joint pain for three years and started taking different drugs but none of them worked. When I had to use a cane to walk I said enough is enough. I made an appointment with Melanie and after two months I'm pain free and can move freely".
Dan Kirpatrick

Let's pause for a moment and look at how far we've come. Our diets include healthy fats and bone broth, our water is clean, we are working out functionally, and we've been applying essential oils to our forehead when we feel a headache coming on. That's impressive. But there is something missing: therapy. While changing your diet and adding functional

> "Most allopathic doctors think practitioners of alternative medicine are all quacks. They're not. Often they're sharp people who think differently about disease." –Dr. Oz

movement can help tremendously, there are a few therapies I recommend to help continue the healing process. Of the many emotional and physical therapies in alternative medicine, I'm mentioning the ones that are most beneficial.

You might have a rheumatologist for arthritis, a cardiologist for a heart condition, and an endocrinologist for low thyroid, but it's time to stop looking at ourselves one organ or system at a time through a specialist's microscope. We are a spirit, with a soul, living in a body. If we are going to recover from an illness we must take on a holistic perspective. Working on body, mind, and spirit accelerates healing. It is when we ignore specific aspects of ourselves that symptoms and conditions continue unchecked. We may stop smoking and quit eating junk food, but we can't forget about the "silent inflammation." Dr. Schneider writes about this in his book. On his journey to weight loss, he wore his body out changing the physical aspects to his problem while completely ignoring the emotional and deep rooted aspects of himself. Despite the weight loss, his health worsened. [67] You and I are the same way. If we ignore our trapped emotions or our negative thinking we will not be in optimal health. We cannot compartmentalize our health thinking that finding a great chiropractor or far infrared sauna will heal us in drive-thru fashion. Rather, each intervention must work holistically to build us up.

With multiple medical specialties, there is often "friendly fire." What does the military definition of accidentally shooting allies have to do with health? Often we want an immediate, powerful solution to a single symptom regardless of the consequences. For example, if we take an antacid or proton pump inhibitor for heartburn, it is also lowering our stomach acid which decreases mineral absorption and may weaken our bones. [96, 97] With the right team of practitioners, there is no friendly fire in natural medicine.

Whether the practitioner is a medical doctor or an alternative health specialist, the holistic approach doesn't sacrifice one organ or symptom for another. Be wary of practitioners who will prescribe so many supplements and therapies that it's hard to remember what your initial problem was. Use them for their special knowledge and skills. A personal trainer isn't the specialist with whom you should discuss genetic disorders, and some physicians have less knowledge about healthy eating than a nutritionist. The concepts of complementary and alternative medicine aren't something that a Western medicine practitioner can quickly grasp at a conference or seminar.

Choosing the Right Health Care Provider for You

Living a natural lifestyle is easier with a health care practitioner who understands, supports, and prescribes in step with your values. Almost half of Americans already implement some form of complimentary alternative medicine to stay healthy and active. Each practitioner offers a unique perspective and your goal is to find a practitioner you deem trustworthy and experienced. The best choice depends upon your individual health needs. There are many health care practitioners that may be of benefit to you from naturopathic doctors to holistic health consultants and even herbalists. For a primary care provider, locate a practitioner who is integrative and can order and interpret lab results plus recommend specific supplements and lifestyle changes to address your needs.

Those needs differ widely, as some people may only need to add a health coach or trainer to encourage them. To manage complex medical problems, you will want to see a functional medicine practitioner or physician who has an integrative approach. If you are looking for suggestions on how to lose weight or manage less serious conditions, there is a wide array of practitioners to choose from. Ask questions, especially about their training and background. What is their degree and are they licensed or certified? I recommend seeing a practitioner with at least two years of experience and client testimonials relatable to your situation. Find out who your friends are seeing. Finally, seek someone you can partner with. My clients find me because they aren't feeling heard or understood by their current practitioner. Search for someone who takes your symptoms seriously and inspires you to live healthier. This will probably take longer than the 15-minute physician appointments you're used to.

Although many of the therapies in this chapter require seeking out an expert, some can be done in the comfort of your own home. First up is a closer look at some relaxing and cleansing therapies, followed by manual interventions such as chiropractic care. Then we'll go a little deeper into alternative medicine and discuss acupuncture, and other meridian clearing modalities. We'll finish with spirituality and a focus on emotional release work.

> *"Melanie was God sent! My daughter came to Melanie in terrible shape coming down from depression/anxiety medication that about killed her. She couldn't sleep, was having involuntary muscle spasms, and had anxiety through the roof. After exposing food allergies, eliminating the foods, adding supplements to support her adrenals, treating a virus, and finding out a very key root of her problems through saliva testing and treating it, she's like a different person. Melanie cares so much for her clients. You can be so discouraged when you come in and be so encouraged when you leave. She never gives up on you! She was an answer to our prayers! My daughter was also diagnosed with scoliosis at age 12 with a 26 and 28 degree curve in her spine. We went to the orthopedic doctor and they put her in a hard and rigid Charleston brace. It was so tight on her that she couldn't breathe, she couldn't sleep with it on, and it was pushing up into her armpit on one side. We turned to chiropractic care and massage. Our chiropractor has been trained in the Schroth Method. After one year of constant chiropractic care and massage therapy, her top curve got better by 2 degrees. The orthopedic doctor had told us the curves would never get better and considered it a success if the curves only got 5 degrees worse with wearing the brace. Every child is different; however, this is what worked for mine and was a huge success. It was truly an answer to our prayers!" Debby Mikayla Parkin*

The Most Important Therapy

Before we summarize therapies requiring qualified practitioners, let's talk about one therapy that trumps them all. Without this one aspect of self-care you may as well forget the rest of the chapter. Some of you may have guessed that I'm already talking about sleep. Yes, it's that important.

Researchers know that the stress hormone cortisol quickly rises when you wake up and gradually tapers as the day goes on, and that a change in this response links to an incredible amount of negative outcomes. In one particular study, the scientists traced cortisol the same way I do for my clients, with multi-day saliva lab work. When they studied daily stress, anticipatory stress, and subjectively reported sleep compared to the cortisol awakening response, they realized that sleep was the key factor and that not enough of it caused cortisol levels to skyrocket. I can't look at your hormone levels in isolation without asking simple questions like how much you slept last night.[98] Sleep is critical to hormone function. Add caffeine to the mix and your body can't remember what it's supposed to do.[99]

There are many methods to help you get a better night's rest, but having to take a pill or supplement long term to help you fall asleep or stay asleep is not a long-term solution, no matter how natural the remedy. These things can be used short term to bring balance, but ultimately you should be able to fall asleep and stay asleep. Ask the majority of Americans and few people have uninterrupted or restful sleep. It is important just like with any other symptom to figure out what is causing your sleep to be disturbed. Is it elevated nighttime cortisol keeping you up? Is it a drop in blood sugar in the middle of the night that wakes you up? Or maybe you wake between 1:00 and 3:00 AM as your liver struggles through phase one or two of detoxification? Whatever the reason, not being able to sleep needs to be addressed. So what can you do to help get a good night's rest?

First, get your hormones tested. Determine whether or not you have high cortisol and work with a skilled practitioner to solve that issue first. A spike in cortisol can happen at any time throughout the day; even a mid-afternoon spike can affect how easily you fall asleep. Seriphos is a great supplement to take when high cortisol is noted. Although we hear a lot about high cortisol, those with low cortisol can have trouble sleeping as well and it is often related to an imbalance in blood sugar. Eating regularly throughout the day, plus a snack before bed, along with supplemental licorice root extract can help boost cortisol if it's too low. Don't forget to have your melatonin levels checked to rule out low levels.

Second, take care of your nervous system. This can be done easily by getting a chiropractic adjustment and avoiding unnecessary electricity at night. I noticed while working in a chiropractor's office that many people reported sleeping so much better after they had an adjustment. We'll talk more about the benefits of chiropractic care a little later. If you are always connected with technology, the evening is a great time to take a break. Prepare for bed at least two hours before sleeping by shutting off the Wi-Fi in your home or at least dimming the screens on your computer and mobile devices. Another option would be to wear the glasses that author Caitlyn Weeks from Grass Fed Girl recommends to filter the light so it won't affect melatonin production.[100]

Lastly, most people are deficient in magnesium. Magnesium is very calming and works well as a sleep aid. It keeps our bones strong and assists with over 300 enzyme reactions in the body. Magnesium can also help with muscular tightness and pain. There are many ways to incorporate magnesium in your daily routine. Among my favorites are an Epsom salt bath or a Natural Calm magnesium drink. Even taking magnesium in supplement form is a positive habit. Magnesium can be found in some foods, but most of us need to supplement our intake because of soil depletion. By increasing magnesium intake, you are building into your daily diet little moments of stress reduction. If you choose to supplement magnesium, always use a bioavailable form such as magnesium malate or magnesium glycinate. It's a good idea to have your magnesium levels checked. The most accurate test is the MAG RBC blood test—6.0 or higher is optimal. To determine the right dose of magnesium, take five times your body weight in magnesium (e.g. if you weigh 100 pounds, take 500 milligrams.). Another easy way to include more magnesium is by using a topically applied magnesium oil or lotion. Transdermal application is often absorbed better than oral supplementation. If you would like to look further at how to easily build up your magnesium, check out gotmag. org or look in this book's recipe section for my favorite magnesium cocktail! Just promise to serve it in a pretty glass.

Colon Care

Colon cleansing has been practiced for more than three thousand years. As early as 1500 B.C., the *Ebers Papyrus*, an ancient Egyptian medical document, described

> "All disease begins in the gut." –Hippocrates

the many benefits of colon cleansing. Until approximately 70 years ago, medical doctors frequently prescribed such cleanses as part of routine treatment for various diseases. Physicians recommended enemas to bring down a fever. Today, medical professionals have little to no training in the value of colon cleansing. Disease begins in the intestines, but health starts there as well. Cleansing is a basic principle in holistic health care and is one secret to a long, healthy, disease-free life.

You may wonder why someone would voluntarily cleanse their colon. The topic may be one you want to avoid altogether, but colon care and cleansing are critical to healing and keeping your body healthy. When waste cannot be properly eliminated, it accumulates in the colon and backs up the rest of the digestive tract, ultimately affecting the liver and kidneys. This waste on the walls of the colon becomes the perfect breeding ground for parasites, yeast, and viruses. The way most of us eat today, toxins will accumulate in our body and it all starts in the digestive tract. Symptoms such as constipation, diarrhea, headaches, weight gain, skin problems, joint pain, depression, premature ageing, and other serious illnesses can all lead to a toxic colon.

Our digestive system is similar to the root system of a tree. Trees take in nutrients and water through their roots, feeding all the branches and leaves. Our root system in essence is our digestive tract, where nutrients from food are carried into our blood stream then passed to various tissues and organs. If there is a blockage or poor nutrient absorption, the entire system is thrown out of balance.

Even for those in reasonably good health, the typical adult digestive tract has worked hard to turn food into nutrients. If you do have a health problem, your digestive tract unquestionably is in poor health. An initial colon cleanse followed by restoring your inner ecosystem with probiotic-rich and nourishing foods can have a dramatic impact on your health. Talk to your health provider first, though. I'll never forget when my natural doctor told me I needed to do an enema!

"There's no way!" I said. It took me over a year to finally do one, and after the experience I wished I would have cleansed my colon sooner. I definitely would have gotten better faster. We recognize the importance of cleaning out our houses and our cars' engines—why not take care of our bodies just as well? Below I'll explain three simple ways to cleanse your colon. The home enema is easy to do and can be tailored to your specific health needs. Colonics can be done by seeing a certified colon hydrotherapist. Lastly, herbs can play a role in colon cleansing, especially if the idea of colonics leaves you squeamish.

Enemas

When administered correctly, enemas are safe, painless, and sanitary. Enemas are used in hospitals when patients are really stopped up, but they serve a purpose to get rid of gut and systemic toxins too. There are two types of enemas: retention and cleansing. Coffee enemas are also considered a retention enema. A study measuring antioxidants didn't find a difference between subjects who drank coffee and those who received it in enema form. [101] I hope the volunteers who received enemas instead of free coffee to drink were compensated generously! Although it doesn't make you jittery when you absorb it in enema form, caffeine stimulates the bile duct to release toxins from the liver into the intestines for removal. This decreases the upregulation (hard work) of liver enzymes associated with pollutants, alcohol, prescription drugs, and anything else requiring extensive metabolism. Unlike colon hydrotherapy, only a small amount of coffee that stays in the sigmoid colon is needed. [102] Always use organic coffee, and check out sawilsons.com for further coffee enema instructions.

A cleansing enema is not retained or held in the body for long time periods. They are mostly used to rinse out the colon. I suggest using filtered water and an enema bag (found at most drug stores and often called a water bottle combination kit). With a cleansing enema, you can add minerals, herbal teas, and even probiotics to the water, which can be very therapeutic. Check out the Home Enemas article on bodyecology.com more information on different types of enemas and more detailed instructions.

Colonics

If you feel unsure about doing an enema at home, consider seeing a colon hydrotherapist in your area. They have professional equipment and facilities to make colon cleansing spa like. Colonic irrigation bathes the entire length of the colon with about 10 gallons of water per session. When administered correctly, colonics are safe, painless, and sanitary. Find an experienced therapist you feel comfortable with and who uses disposable tubing and attachments.

Colon cleansing will help your liver as well as lymphatic system. Once your colon is free of blockages, colonics, and enemas can be used whenever you are ill or when "cleansing." Colon cleansing will not wash away beneficial microflora since they are safely tucked into the intestinal lining. After colon cleansing, always recolonize your colon by taking probiotics supplements orally or by eating probiotic-rich foods such as cultured vegetables and kefir.

Cleansing Herbs

There are many herbs and foods that are cleansing. Simply using garlic in your cooking or eating salads with cultured vegetables can enhance digestion. Herbs such as aloe, senna, and cascara sagrada act as laxatives. They can be used occasionally, but only for a short period of time. Colon cleansing products often contain psyllium or bentonite clay. When consuming any cleansing herbs or foods, drink plenty of water as these products have considerable amounts of fiber.

Physical Therapy

Many similar practices derive much of their philosophy from physical manipulation of the body. This chapter isn't meant to be an alternative health encyclopedia, but rather an introduction into helpful therapies along your journey to wellness.

Chiropractic (and Osteopathy)

Chiropractors believe our bodies can heal themselves when the skeletal system is in proper alignment and the nervous system is functioning optimally. A chiropractor will adjust the spine with his or her hands or an adjustment tool in order to treat subluxation. When the spine is out of alignment because of subluxation, nerve transmissions are disrupted, causing pain and potentially other illnesses throughout the body. Contrary to what many believe, chiropractic care is not just for those with back pain. Patients with various types of headaches and even those with ADD/ADHD, chronic diarrhea, and other seemingly unrelated issues also report relief. [103] **Craniosacral manipulation** is a similar technique used by osteopaths.

Spinal manipulation has been around for centuries, but the father of modern chiropractic care is Daniel Palmer. Palmer believed that all communication from the brain to the rest of the body went through the spinal canal. If any area of the spinal canal was stressed or out of alignment, uncomfortable physical symptoms could arise. In the United States, chiropractic care is gaining widespread use for its ability to allow patients to heal chronic problems often without using medicine. Although chiropractic is a natural practice, the medical field is more open to this specialty due to scientific evidence and the clear correlation of our spinal cord to the rest of our bodies. Chiropractic care combines alternative and conventional medicine and offers very few risks in the hands of a competent practitioner. Search for a chiropractor the same way you would a physician, keeping in mind word of mouth from trusted friends often works best.

The most common side effect is slight discomfort in the area adjusted. Because of their muscle-relaxing properties, essential oils such as frankincense help patients "hold" their adjustments longer between sessions. Some practitioners attribute this to the high-energy frequency in these oils, and studies show physical differences in smooth and skeletal muscle attributed to various oil blends. [104]

A patient should be referred to a medical doctor if despite the best in chiropractic care, the pain continues or a deformity needs more serious care such as surgery. Although studies show reduced low back pain and disability with chiropractic care, it's important to note that the individual practitioner matters. [105] There are several other traditional medical approaches, especially surgery, that cost more than chiropractic care, and they're not necessarily more effective in acute and chronic back pain patients. [106, 107] I visited several chiropractors before I found one my spine enjoyed being around. One chiropractor's office had a waterbed therapy table that broke while I was on it, soaking me before I headed off to work.

Massage Therapy

I always thought massage therapy was a luxury and didn't realize how beneficial it can be. Years ago when I lived in Ohio, my chiropractor recommended that I see a massage therapist. It was then that I learned that massage needs the word therapy behind it. Not only is massage therapy relaxing, it also keeps the lymphatic system flowing and lowers cortisol. Deep tissue is a favorite of mine when I've been at the computer too long or chopping at the cutting board and my elbows start to hurt. It's not the aspirin I reach for; it's the phone to make an appointment. After doing massage therapy regularly for over nine years, I am rarely in pain, and if I am, I know where I need to go.

> I had residual arm pain from a car accident that massage therapy and chiropractic care were not addressing. After one session of Rolfing in Pensacola with Sharalee Hoelscher, the pain was completely gone.

My friend Brandi, a licensed massage therapist whom I interviewed for *The Nourishing Podcast*, mentions how preventative massage therapy can be: it's not just for pain, but general toning and conditioning, too. Some massage therapists have specialties such as cupping, Rolfing, acupressure, or reflexology. Most massage therapists can tailor the appointment to include what is needed at the time. Rolfing is a massage technique meant to reorganize connective tissue. Briefly, cupping follows the Eastern tradition of drawing blood to an area via suction to promote healing. One of my clients states that cupping is the only therapy that relieves her back pain. As any massage therapist will tell you, drink up after a massage because the therapy can kick up some toxins.

Acupressure

Many years ago, a massage therapist taught me basic acupressure during a session. Imagine our body as several freeway systems covering us from head to toe. Sometimes along these "freeways" or meridians there can be little car accidents blocking the flow of traffic. It could be from stress, a food allergy, a hormone imbalance, whatever, but for whatever reason the energy is blocked. Our amazing bodies were designed intricately, and in many cases we can heal ourselves. Keeping with the same theme, many massage therapists also do reflexology, which is acupressure but just on the feet. Various regions on the foot were mapped by the Chinese and Egyptians thousands of years ago to affect healing in all the organs of the body. For most people, letting someone massage their feet is an easier step than accepting the needles of an acupuncturist, especially since Eastern medical philosophies are so unique. Let's continue learning about this freeway system in our bodies and how acupuncture can help.

Acupuncture

Many of the concepts emphasized in traditional Chinese medicine have no true counterpart in Western medicine. What happens to one part of the body affects every other part. The mind and body are not viewed separately, but as part of an energetic system. Organs and organ systems are viewed as interconnected structures that work together to keep the body functioning. Energy flows through the body via 20 channels called **meridians**. These pathways are primary or secondary and correspond to specific organs or functions. Imbalances in the flow of energy can cause illness until correct flow restores the body to balance. While acupuncture is the most often practiced component of traditional Chinese medicine, it is simply that—a component, an important piece of a much larger puzzle.

NAET/Bioset (Modern Meridian Systems)

Dr. Nadrumipad created a system of allergy clearing called NAET, which stands for Nadrumipad's Allergy Elimination Technique. NAET is a form of acupressure that works with the immune and nervous system to help alleviate symptoms associated with many health conditions, but I find it especially helpful in autoimmune cases. There are more than 80 different types of autoimmune disorders affecting 50 million people in the United States. [108]

Earlier we discussed our body being a freeway of meridians, when NAET is performed or the similar system Bioset, it clears the meridian system that is causing the symptoms. [109] It's almost as if we have the opportunity to retrain the immune system and nervous system to know what to attack and what not to attack. I find these systems work best in people who are simultaneously healing their gut and avoiding potential toxins and electromagnetic fields. [110] Bioset is based on the work of Dr. Elaine Cutler and her book *The Food Allergy Cure: A New Solution to Food Cravings, Obesity, Depression, Headaches, Arthritis, and Fatigue.* In a non-allergenic nutshell, Elaine Cutler's method uses immunology, electromagnetic wave research, detoxification, enzyme therapy, and nutrition.

One aspect of functional medicine I adore is its ability to personalize natural health to the individual. There are many herbs and supplements available, but without a targeted approach, it's unlikely that a bottle randomly pulled from the vitamin store shelf will turn someone's health around. Yet another chiropractic technique that incorporates all these systems is applied **kinesiology**, or muscle testing. The best format for this kind of diagnostic work comes from Nutrition Response Testing (SM), the revolutionary system based on the above research and developed by chiropractor Freddy Ulan after years of clinical study and thousands of **case studies**.

Nutrition Response Testing uses simple reflexes to test for autonomic nervous system dysfunction. Organs are said to be "weak" or "strong" depending on limb strength in response to supportive supplements. Evidence shows that the autonomic nervous system is the correct place to target for this kind of therapy, which is distantly related to psychoneuroimmunological mediation. I won't mention that again though—too many letters. Basically, the autonomic nervous system innervates every complex connection in the body without any conscious control on our part. Autonomic nervous system activity is altered by the chiropractic and meridian therapies I've just mentioned. In one study, 55% of patients found these therapies to be very helpful. The 55% also includes patients who only chose guided imagery to help them with arthritis and digestive issues. [111]

> I explain the autonomic nervous system here: http://www.ehow.com/video_12305742_teaching-stategies-nervous-system.html

Emotional Release Work

In comparison to some of the techniques I've mentioned and the ones I'm going to discuss here, homeopathic remedies may resemble standard medical care. However, this book would be incomplete if I didn't mention some of the unconventional therapies that I still use to improve my health and make a marked difference for my clients. Some of these techniques have been used for thousands of years and are further bolstered by **double-blinded research** studies to prove their efficacy, while others are mostly backed by anecdotal evidence and differ widely from practitioner to practitioner. As a quick review, "I lost 15 pounds in two days with this wonder shake!" is also anecdotal evidence. It's true for that person, but the average person may not achieve the same results. I originally planned to include a list of energy therapies that are completely ludicrous and won't help anyone, but that blurry continuum from fraud to fantastic is just too fragile to make definitive statements.

Studies have shown that emotional release work and even **energy medicine** reduce anxiety and pain, relax muscles, and promote wound healing, but more definitive research is needed. [112] Most practitioners will assure you that patients from any religion or belief system can undergo therapy without a problem. As a Christian, I avoid any mind-altering therapies because I want to always be in charge of my faculties and understand what's going on. The therapies I'm discussing incorporate multiple therapies and holistic techniques. There is a reason I've also chosen to discuss emotions and spirituality in this chapter. I have a specific stance on energy healing and alternative therapies that you may or may not agree with. I believe that all healing energy comes from God, who created the medicine, had the knowledge, or created the remedy for use in the first place (Psalm 24:1).

> The individual relationship between the practitioner and the client is important, and without trust and understanding on a spiritual level you're unlikely to find healing from this branch of natural medicine.

I'll also avoid anything that makes me hesitate and feel uneasy (Romans 14:23). The individual relationship between the practitioner and the client is important, and without trust and understanding on a spiritual level you're unlikely to find healing from this branch of natural medicine. You simply need to know what you're getting into and how it aligns with your personal philosophy of how the world works.

Emotions are Powerful.

Our emotions and thoughts can be a very powerful catalyst for a quick healing or a slow and long process to delayed healing. As I detail in a few paragraphs, scientists are discovering that our thoughts affect genes. Studies show that it's not our conscious thoughts or affirmations that are the most powerful. It's the subconscious thoughts.

Emotions and feelings that we aren't even aware of influence our health and wellbeing. In traditional Chinese medicine, emotions or feelings that we don't process or are recurring can get trapped in an organ or become a part of our nervous system. As an example, the kidneys are associated with fear, and the gallbladder is often associated with frustration.

Emotions can influence us exactly the same way as a food sensitivity or chemical toxicity. Trapped or negative emotions are inflammatory in nature and can wreak havoc. You may have heard that a cheerful heart is good medicine, and it's true. So what can we do with negative emotions, or better yet, subconscious emotions? The first place to start is forgiveness. True emotional release work all comes down to forgiving ourselves and forgiving those who have hurt us. It really is time to let it go. When we become upset with someone and we hold it in and carry bitterness for months or even years, it has no effect on the other person, just us. I've seen some amazing things happen when buried emotions are released and healthy emotions take their place.

One tool I use with my clients is the book *Releasing Emotional Patterns with Essential Oils*. Author Carolyn L. Mein D.C. shows you how to determine your body type and then which organs have the potential for trapped emotions. This is a great first step, especially for subconscious attitudes and emotions. Mein offers specific phrases to state while applying the oil to a specific acupressure point. It's a novel idea, but the results I have seen with this type of therapy on myself and my clients are nothing short of astounding. Afterwards, most people feel as though they can breathe deeper and that circumstances that used to upset them don't bother them anymore. Repeat the process to release subconscious emotions as needed.

Studies at the University of Edinburgh show that the amygdala (the limbic system gland that stores and releases trauma in the body) does not respond to sound, sight or touch. It only releases trauma through aromatic stimuli, the sense of smell. [113] Breathing in essential oils has a powerful effect on releasing emotions.

Emotions and Disease

Remember the functional medicine pathway in Chapter Three? It's one of the only pictures in this book and diagrams how medical diagnoses can start as simple imbalances. Our emotions are similar. Surface anxieties and behaviors intertwine with complex physical symptoms fed from underneath the surface. The roots can be bitterness or legitimate physiological problems but they are rarely exposed so we can dig them out and deal with them. I can treat a client's Candida or food allergy or acne all day time after time, but sometimes the key has been a more abstract problem like unforgiveness, lack of acceptance, or a longing heart.

If you don't think this is a problem, research how antidepressant drugs are prescribed to alleviate cancer pain or how drugs that work on the mind like Neurontin and Lyrica are a main treatment for fibromyalgia and other poorly understood pain syndromes. We need to learn how to deal with emotions. Unsettled emotions are devastating to the mind, body, and soul, whether you are a professional athlete needing to be on top of your physical game, like my friend Junior DeSouza, or simply struggle with the frenetic pace of life here in America. I don't just want to pick on pain and fibromyalgia either—that's too easy, everyone does that, and I don't want to start a conversation about psychosomatic versus "real" pain. Researchers tested women with another autoimmune disease, lupus, to see if their symptoms and vulnerability to the disease related to emotional connectedness and control. The short answer is "yes." They were tested on emotional attachment and the ability to understand and describe their own attitudes and emotions. Not surprisingly, the women tested highly for an unresolved and entangled state of mind. Their inability to recognize and fully experience their own emotions seemed to be a defensive way to avoid painful memories. Besides impeding their clinical progress, this detachment also affected their abilities to meaningfully attach with others. [114]

The Effect of Mind and Emotion on Genes

New studies are now confirming the connection between emotions, genes, and the importance of sleep. I traced this and similar research back to the February 2014 volume of *Psychoneuroendocrinology*. The study started with two groups engaged in quiet activities. The study group meditated on mindfulness while the control group did not. Mindfulness is the exact opposite of checking texts and eating kale chips while you're reading this book. Rather, I define it as a purposeful, calming focus on the present, on current feelings rather than plans for the future or influences from the past. After eight hours, the meditators showed a range of genetic and molecular differences, including altered levels of gene-regulating laboratory values and reduced levels of pro-inflammatory genes, which in turn correlated with faster physical recovery from a stressful situation. The genes included cortisol secretors and **COX inhibitors**, which play a pivotal role in inflammation. These differences were not present in pre-study testing, so it's safe to say the changes were due to the differences in how the two groups spent their eight hours of quiet activity.[115]

Quiet moments aren't the only ones ripe for mindfulness. My husband and I were watching the television finale of one of those sing and dance competitions. As is customary for such shows, they had a teenage heartthrob, irrelevant to large swaths of society, perform several feet away from an adoring audience. The camera panned to show his hordes of screaming female fans, and none of them were looking at him—not a single one. They could have tackled him for a hug, but instead they were all texting their friends or preparing to take the best selfie of the year. His fans were trying to record memories and let their friends know about their newfound prestige rather than be there live, in the moment, connecting face to face with their idol.

Altering perception and focus can create thousands of variations in each gene just by changes in blood chemistry. This correlates with research showing that your beliefs about how healthy a food is, changes your secretion of appetite and digestive hormones. The researchers compared it to the nocebo (opposite of placebo) effect of hearing you have six months to live and dying in six months regardless of disease progression. For a less morbid example, research shows that pituitary hormones and the autonomic nervous system activate when someone expects to get better, even if it's just a placebo effect. [111]

This news about the power of the mind is great, right? Let's just say some positive affirmations, incorporate Eastern mysticism, throw in some fervent prayers to Jesus, and we'll cover all our bases. Not quite! You see, all this stuff is subconscious. One of the study authors explained that our mind bridges beliefs and reality and adjusts biology and behavior to fit our faith. This is why those with multiple personalities and similar dissociative disorders can have food allergies or other physical problems that disappear when another personality manifests. We can't just think our way to good health. We have to believe it inside and out.

Spiritual

The last few techniques I'm advocating blur the lines between positive thinking, spirituality, and emotions. Let me illustrate my point with a fascinating study that connects us back to the chapter about fat, sugar, and how our beliefs shape our ability to lose weight and thrive. It's always been a mystery to me how some people can do so well on controversial diets that I assumed wouldn't impact anyone's health, but it all has to do with the placebo effect. Researchers made a batch of milkshakes but slapped one of two possible labels on them. One advertised the product as a sensible, reduced-fat, reduced-sugar, and reduced-calorie shake, while the other label emphasized what a rich and decadent treat the milkshake was. Both labels were incorrect, but researchers drew lab values of ghrelin to see if beliefs can change physiology. Similar to leptin, ghrelin is a satiety peptide with widespread receptors. It reinforces addictive eating behaviors, but it is useful for telling you when to eat and how much. Researchers discovered that ghrelin levels were highest in both groups right before ingesting the shakes, just as they expected. However, after drinking the shakes, ghrelin levels dropped off much more dramatically in the group who thought they had just finished a sinful treat. Ghrelin levels are supposed to drop off after a satisfying meal, but they barely budged in the group with the "diet" shake.[116]

> Chemical and physiological reactions in your gut triggered by the composition of the substances you ingest are no match for the emotions and values you attach to your actions.

That's how powerful your beliefs are. Chemical and physiological reactions in your gut triggered by the composition of the substances you ingest are no match for the emotions and values you attach to your actions. Simply put, thoughts affect digestion. As I mentioned in the first chapter, praying and connecting with God played a vital role in my path to wellness. I maintained a "spiritual detox" to keep my focus and emotions uncluttered from guilt, bitterness, envy, and those other swirling emotions that occurred all too readily when I struggled to just digest a meal. Everyone around seemed to be in perfect health but no one could explain what was wrong with my body. I prayed healing scripture verses over my life and learned the importance of positive confessions, affirmations, and hope. Your personal beliefs as well as your ability to have faith and not lose hope are some of the most powerful weapons you wield against sickness.

Fasting

Similar to the mindfulness mentioned in the previous section, fasting is a useful spiritual tool. Going without teaches us what we're truly hungry for and improves discernment. Is it carbs? I'm craving, emotional connection with others, or is it my soul that is hungry? I've done many different kinds of fasts, and all have produced physical and spiritual improvement. However, fasting without introspection and a willingness to change just results in hunger. When I fast, I always include prayer and reading the Bible along with dietary changes. This is a powerful combination to restore my soul by allowing God to illuminate emotions or past events that need processing. Proverbs 20:5 says it best: "Counsel in the heart of man is like deep water; but a man of understanding will draw it out." (KJV). Junior Desouza explains that this verse depicts the deepest part of your heart as deep waters. As we learned in the water chapter, water needs filtered to be cleansed. While fasting, past events or emotions may resurface that need dealt with and released. Fasting has the power to break addictions like nothing else (Isaiah 58). Below are a few of the fasts I recommend under the care of a practitioner if your mind and body is ready.

Ten-Day Daniel Fast

The ten-day Daniel fast is a modified fast based upon the biblical Daniel and his Hebrew friends who fasted from rich foods and wine. They primarily ate fruits and vegetables. Other excellent short-term cleanses just eliminate all forms of sugar, caffeine, junk foods, and dairy products. [40] Juice fasting has become very trendy since the movie *Fat, Sick, and Nearly Dead* chronicled the amazing transformation of Australian Joe Cross. Juice fasting involves vegetable juice and water. There is a right and a wrong way to do juice fasts. Before embarking on such a fast, you should already be eating whole foods and have a clean diet—nourishing foods before and after a fast decrease the stress on your body. It's also important to include enemas into an extended juice fast cleansing routine. This type of fast drastically slows down intestinal peristalsis (movement). Do one enema every day of the fast or see a colon hydrotherapist for a colonic. This ensures success because it eliminates cravings. I've done one, three, and five day juice cleanses that were powerfully detoxing. Juice fasting isn't for everyone, especially those with blood sugar issues. I also do not recommend multiple juice fasts as they can affect metabolism negatively.

Bone Broth Fast

Similar to juice fasting is a bone broth fast. On this type of fast, usually three days or less, make soup with organic animal bones—one of my recipes is in the appendix. Your soup can be all vegetable soups or you can add protein. This fast is incredibly gut-healing. Giving your body a break from digesting food is essentially like hitting the reset button.

Water-Only Fast

The last and most powerful fast is a water-only fast. I remember a time in my healing journey where I knew I needed to do this step in order to completely heal my gut. Under the care of my natural doctor, I embarked on a three-day water-only fast. Extended water fasts are not recommended, and certain health conditions make this a very risky option. Juice fasting rules apply. A daily enema allows for optimal detoxification and craving eradication. Water only fasting is an extreme type of fast but it does have benefits such as regulating our immune system and healing our digestive tract.

Prayer, fasting, and relaxation are formidable ways to improve your health, whether you visit a practitioner or practice ways to release stress at home or work. Countless studies show the benefits of all these approaches, but one of my favorites involved congestive heart failure patients because that particular disease is the epitome of stress—a feebly beating heart can't keep up with the oxygen demands of tissues and fluid imbalances that threaten to swell up ankles at best and drown lungs at worst. Every cell is in survival mode during congestive heart failure, but researchers taught 20-minute relaxation techniques to

Action Step: Learn from the experts.

Go to thegreciangarden.com/podcast or type **The Nourishing Podcast** into iTunes or your favorite podcast player. You'll find episodes where my co-host Emily and I talk to natural practitioners and therapists to discover which therapy is just perfect to add to your wellness plan.

Action Step: The perfect way to end your day.
Make a Magnesium Cocktail. A great recipe can be found in the appendix.

these patients. Over half of them got better and also reported healthy lifestyle changes and better relationships with others. [117]

Continuing the Journey

It's like this. When I was sick, it was a real struggle to even make the decision of where to turn next. Should I swallow the anti-fungal prescription from the integrative medicine doctor, take a break and exist on Styrofoam-flavored rice crackers, or just curl up in the fetal position and pray? I wouldn't be in the position I am today if I hadn't realized that I also needed to be healed emotionally and spiritually if I expected a turnaround. Really, that's what this book is about. Learn yourself. Study your digestive patterns. Learn what foods nourish, satiate, and energize you. Ignore anything I've said that doesn't apply to your situation, and embrace the changes that will propel you on the path to wellness, whether it's a new exercise, alternative therapy, or even a new perspective on life and the importance of your beliefs and emotions. It's all connected. We can use "holistic," "integrative," "synergistic," and every other handy buzz word, but it needs to resonate deeply within that we are not compartmentalized beings. There are no walls.

A solution has emerged to help with the growing burden of chronic disease. It derives from the approach that we are all unique and there is no one size fits all therapy. The question is: How will you adjust your lifestyle, diet, and environment to best suit your health goals? I've presented several tools to help personalize progress by adjusting your diet and improving your physical movement. I've also included a resource section at the end of the book with key websites on obtaining your own lab work and how to find various practitioners. I hope it leads you to make positive changes. I know that it's not easy and that even the philosophy of constantly needing to change one more thing to reach wellness is not healthy. Think of what you've read here as guidelines and suggestions rather than a book of rules and algorithms leading to perfection.

But what if you understand yourself perfectly but still can't find the solution? Don't give up! Find a trained practitioner who will work with you to uncover what root causes are potentially not yet addressed. As you've hopefully noticed, my goal with this book is not the absurd idea that I could offer the exact, individual information for every single person who reads it. Rather, it's that each and every one of you will take a hard look at habits, beliefs, or symptoms, and accept where you need to make changes. I hope I've opened up a world of opportunities, a path to wellness, and a sense of hope.

Appendix

Appendix A: MTHFR Gene Expression Possibilities

List updated: December 6, 2012

Autism	Chemical sensitivity
Addictions: smoking, drugs, alcohol	Colorectal adenoma
	Idiopathic male infertility
Down's syndrome	Blood clots
Miscarriages	Rectal cancer
Pulmonary embolisms	Meningioma
Depression in post-menopausal women	Glioma
	Congenital heart defects
Schizophrenia	Infant depression via epigenetic
Fibromyalgia	processes caused by maternal
Chronic fatigue syndrome	depression
Chemical sensitivity	Deficits in childhood cognitive
Parkinson's	development
Irritable bowel syndrome	Gastric cancer
Pre-eclampsia	Migraines with aura
Stroke	Low HDL
Spina bifida	High homocysteine
Esophageal squamous cell Carcinoma	Post-menopausal breast cancer
	Atherosclerosis
Acute lymphoblastic leukemia	Oral clefts
Vascular dementia	Type 1 diabetes
Bipolar disorder	Cervical dysplasia
Epilepsy	Increased bone fracture risk in
Primary closed-angle glaucoma	post-menopausal women
Alzheimer's	Multiple sclerosis
Tetralogy of tallot	Essential hypertension
Decreased telomere length	Differentiated thyroid carcinoma
Potential drug toxicities: methotrexate, anti-epileptics	Prostate cancer

Appendix B: How do I change to a healthier diet?
Start with the easiest transition.

If you feel overwhelmed, that's ok. It takes time to change and learn new habits. View the chart below and select the foods you can upgrade and use.

Standard	Healthier substitute (Real Food)
Mac and cheese with hot dogs	Rice penne and pesto with chicken sausages
Frozen pizza	Homemade pizza using bruschetta topped with eggplant and turkey pepperoni (optional)
Peanut butter and jelly	Almond butter with jam on sprouted grain bread
Potato chips	Nori chips or kale chips
Store-bought dip	Easy homemade guacamole
Egg Mcmuffin	Baked eggs with green onions, spinach, and dill

Appendix C: Soy

Cultures including soy in their diet have traditionally eaten it in a fermented form, such as natto or soy sauce. This removes phytic acid and enzyme inhibitors to ensure that soy remains digestible and nourishing. High levels of phytic acid in soy block absorption of calcium, magnesium, copper, iron, and zinc. Unlike other legumes, phytic acid in soy is not neutralized by ordinary preparation methods such as soaking, sprouting and long, slow cooking. High-phytate diets and trypsin inhibitors in soy interfere with children's growth.

Soy phytoestrogens alter endocrine function and possibly increase infertility, breast and thyroid cancer, and hypothyroidism rates in adult women. Soy formula has been linked to autoimmune thyroid issues in infants. Improperly prepared soy increased the body's requirement for vitamins B12 and D. Finally, processing soy releases the neurotoxin and appetite stimulator MSG. [118-121]

Appendix D: Environmental Working Group's
Clean 15 and Dirty Dozen Lists

Clean Fifteen	Dirty Dozen
Asparagus	Apples
Avocados	Celery
Cabbage	Cherry tomatoes
Cantaloupe	Cucumbers
Cauliflower	Grapes
Eggplant	Nectarines
Grapefruit	Peaches
Kiwi fruit	Potatoes
Mango	Snap peas
Onions	Spinach
Papayas	Strawberries
Pineapples	Sweet bell peppers
Sweet corn	+ hot peppers, kale/collard greens
Sweet peas	
Sweet potatoes	

http://www.ewg.org/foodnews/?gclid=COv459qd-8UCFVMX
HwodqBEAmQ, 2015 list

Recipes

Elderberry syrup

Ingredients

½ cup dried elderberries (or 1 cup fresh)

3 cups water

½ cup raw honey

¼ cup cherry brandy (optional)

Directions

1. Bring to boil dried elderberries (or fresh) in water for 20 minutes. Strain.
2. Add the liquid back to the heat and reduce to 1 cup of liquid. Add raw honey and cherry brandy (optional).
3. Stir well and store in the fridge for up to six months.

Take 1-2 tsp daily for prevention, and 3-5 tsp spread out over the day when sickness comes a-knocking. You can even give this every morning to the kids. If you would like a visual of how to make tinctures and other herbal medicines, check out my video series on Natural Medicine and Health Products (http://www.ehow.com/video_12305740_herbal-preparation-medicinal-plants.html)

Gluten-Free Sourdough Blueberry Muffins

I know what you are thinking, "So what, blueberry muffins? I can make those with my eyes closed." These baby blues are a totally different creature from the blueberry muffins of yesteryear. The beauties we make are much healthier than your standard muffin because I'm showing you how to soak and ferment the grains, which allows their nutrients to be easily broken down and absorbed.

Ingredients

1 cup mature gluten free levain starter culture
1 cup brown rice flour (or your favorite whole grain blend)
½ cup water or whey
¼ tsp salt
1 tsp baking soda
¼ cup coconut palm sugar
½ cup arrowroot starch
½ tsp ground cinnamon
1 egg
If vegan, substitute 1 flax egg.
1 tsp vanilla
¼ cup grapeseed oil, butter, or coconut oil
¾ cup blueberries, fresh or frozen

Directions

1. The night before you plan to make these, combine the starter culture, the brown rice flour, and the water or whey. Stir well and let sit loosely covered overnight.
2. The day you plan to make these, Preheat oven to 425 degrees Fahrenheit and line your muffin tin with cupcake liners.
3. In a large bowl combine the salt, baking soda, palm sugar, cinnamon, and arrowroot starch. Stir in the blueberries.
4. In a small bowl, combine the oil, vanilla, and egg.

5. Combine the starter culture mixture (overnight mixture) with the dry ingredients (blueberries included) in the large bowl. Then mix in the wet ingredients.

6. Spoon the mixture into a prepared muffin pan approximately 3/4 full. Bake at 425 degrees Fahrenheit for 20 minutes or until golden on top and a toothpick inserted in the center comes out clean.

7. Allow them to cool slightly before serving. We spread ours with Kerrygold Irish butter and they were insanely delicious!

Hydration Drink (Homemade Gatorade)

Ingredients

1 cup lemon juice
½ cup honey
1 tsp mineral salt
½ tsp baking soda
Filtered water

Directions

1. Except for water, mix all the ingredients into a bowl and pour into a gallon jug.

2. Fill with water to the top and shake once you put on the lid.

3. Store in refrigerator and drink as needed.

Magnesium Cocktail

For the magnesium drink mix, I use Natural Calm by Natural Vitality or Serine Calm by Source Naturals.

Ingredients

1 cup Rehydration Drink (see Hydration Drink recipe)
½-1 tsp magnesium drink mix
Ice cubes

Directions

1. Pour rehydration drink into a mason jar and add powdered magnesium drink mix.
2. Add in a handful of ice cubes.
3. Put lid on tight, and shake vigorously.
4. Pour drink into cocktail glass, sit back, sip and relax.

Margarita's Baked Salmon with Garlic and Rosemary

Ingredients

5 salmon fillets, boneless (about 1 lb)
1 inch fresh ginger, peeled, chopped, and finely grated
4 cloves garlic, sliced thin
¼ tsp salt
¼ tsp black pepper
¼ cup fresh lemon juice
1 Tbsp fresh rosemary chopped (or 2 tsp dry)

Directions

1. Preheat oven to 375 degrees Fahrenheit. Wash salmon and pat dry. Place in an oiled glass baking dish, drizzle with olive oil, lemon juice and with salt and pepper. Sprinkle on top of salmon the sliced garlic, grated ginger, and rosemary. Drizzle again with olive oil.

2. Bake in the oven covered for 30 minutes and uncovered for 5 minutes.

Mineral-Rich Bone Broth

Ingredients

2 whole free-range chickens (bones, meat removed after roasting)
4 qt filtered water
Juice of one lemon
1 large onion, rough-chopped
2 unpeeled carrots, rough-chopped
3 celery stalks, rough-chopped
2 cloves garlic peeled, rough-chopped

Directions

1. Place chicken bones and all other ingredients into large stock-pot. Let stand for 30 minutes. This step ensures minerals will be transferred from the bones to the broth.
2. Bring to a boil and remove the scum that floats to the top. Reduce heat, cover, and continue simmering for 24 or more hours.
3. When you are finished cooking the stock remove all the chicken parts and vegetables. Pick through chicken bones to remove any remaining meat. Add vegetables to a soup or store in fridge for a side dish. Strain broth into a large bowl and place in refrigerator overnight.
4. At this point, I either make soup or pour the broth into several jars. I keep some jars in the fridge, and put at least one in the freezer for a later use.

Nori Snack recipe

Incorporate seaweed as an easy and healthy lunch or snack on the go. My favorite way to eat seaweed though is toasted sheets of nori that have been seasoned with salt. I eat them just like potato chips. You can also purchase these at the local health food store.

Ingredients

4 sheets toasted nori
Toasted sesame oil
Sea salt

Directions

1. Preheat oven to 250 degrees Fahrenheit.
2. Cut nori into small squares using sharp scissors.
3. Place nori onto cookie sheet and using a pastry brush, brush a light coating of toasted sesame oil onto both the front and backs of the squares.
4. Sprinkle a little sea salt on them.
5. Bake for 15 to 20 minutes. Let cool and place into a container.

Nutrient-Dense Meatloaf

Serves 6-8
Grass-fed liver isn't so bad, especially when you add it to this hearty and healthy meatloaf. Lamb's liver seems the mildest to me. Start with that before trying beef liver.

Ingredients

1 lb grass-fed ground beef
½ lb grass-fed ground liver
Juice from1/2 lemon
2 eggs from pasture raised hens, beaten
½ yellow onion, minced
2 cloves garlic, minced

½ tsp rosemary, crushed

½ tsp cumin

3 Tbsp fresh parsley, minced

1 Tbsp freshly squeezed lemon juice

1 Tbsp coconut oil, melted

Sea salt and ground black pepper to taste

Directions

1. Soak the liver in the juice of half a lemon and filtered water for at least 30 minutes and up to overnight in the fridge.

2. Rinse liver thoroughly and shred with the appropriate food processor attachments, or pulse with a food processor blade until a smooth consistency is reached. Combine liver with all other ingredients and mix together evenly.

3. Press mixture into a glass pan and bake in oven preheated to 375 degrees Fahrenheit for 35 minutes covered and for the last 10 minutes uncovered (45 minutes total) or until the center of your meatloaf is done.

Optional: I have made this recipe with other organ meats as well. Why not try heart?

Citations

CHAPTER 2

1. Mathur, Sonia. "With Diseases, Genetics Loads The Gun and Environment Pulls the Trigger." The Huffington Post Impact Canada. May 8, 2013. www.huffingtonpost.ca/soania-mathur/avoiding-parkinsons-disease_b_3234752.html.

2. Fasano, Alessio. "Leaky Gut and Autoimmune Diseases." *Clinical Reviews in Allergy & Immunology* 42, no. 1 (2012): 71-8.

3. Riediger, Natalie D., Rgia A. Othman, Miyoung Suh, and Mohammed H. Moghadasian. "A Systemic Review of The Roles Of N-3 Fatty Acids In Health And Disease." *Journal of the American Dietetic Association* 109, no. 4 (2009): 668-79.

4. Eswaran, Shanti, Jan Tack, and William Chey. "Food: The Forgotten Factor in the Irritable Bowel Syndrome." *Gastroenterology Clinics* 40, no. 1 (2011).

5. Wahls, Terry L., and Eve Adamson. *The Wahls Protocol: How I Beat Progressive MS Using Paleo Principles and Functional Medicine.* New York: Penguin Group, 2014.

6. Hofmann, Alan F. "Bile Acids: Trying to Understand Their Chemistry and Biology with the Hope of Helping Patients." *Hepatology* 45, no. 9 (2008): 1403-418.

7. Kim, Do Young, Junwei Hao, Ruolan Liu, Gregory Turner, Fu-Dong Shi, and Jong M. Rho. "Inflammation-Mediated

Memory Dysfunction and Effects of a Ketogenic Diet in a Murine Model of Multiple Sclerosis." *PLoS ONE* 7, no. 5 (2012).

8. Taubes, Gary. *Good Calories, Bad Calories: Challenging the Conventional Wisdom on Diet, Weight Control, and Disease.* New York: Knopf, 2007.

9. Keys, Ancel. *Seven Countries: A Multivariate Analysis of Death and Coronary Heart Disease.* Cambridge, Mass.: Harvard University Press, 1980.

10. DeBakey, Michael E., et al. *Journal of the American Medical Association.* (1964).

11. Writing Group for The Women's Health Initiative Investigators, and Jacques Rossouw et al. "Risks and Benefits of Estrogen Plus Progestin in Healthy Postmenopausal Women: Principal Results From the Women's Health Initiative Randomized Controlled Trial." *The Journal of the American Medical Association* 288, no. 3 (2002): 321-33.

12. Appel, Lawrence et al. A Clinical Trial of the Effects of Dietary Patterns on Blood Pressure. *New England Journal of Medicine* 336 (1997): 1117-24.

13. Meyerfreund, Diana, Christine P Gonçalves, Roberto S Cunha, Alexandre C Pereira, José E Krieger, and José G Mill. "Age-dependent Increase in Blood Pressure in Two Different Native American Communities in Brazil." *Journal of Hypertension* 27, no. 9 (2009): 1753-760.

14. Stolarz-Skrzypek, Katarzyna et al. "Fatal and Nonfatal Outcomes, Incidence of Hypertension, and Blood Pressure Changes in Relation to Urinary Sodium Excretion." *The Journal of the American Medical Association* 305, no. 17 (2011): 1777-785.

15. Könner, A. Christine, and Jens C. Brüning. "Selective Insulin and Leptin Resistance in Metabolic Disorders." *Cell Metabolism* 16, no. 2 (2012): 144-52.

CHAPTER 3

16. Bell, Iris, and Mary Koithan. "Models for the Study of Whole Systems." *Integrative Cancer Therapies* 5, no. 4 (2006): 293-307.

17. Ioannidis, John. "Why Most Published Research Findings Are False." *PLoS Medicine* 2, no. 8 (2005): E124. www.plosmedicine.org.

18. Hyman, Mark. "The failure of risk factor treatment for primary prevention of chronic disease." *Alternative Therapies in Health and Medicine* 16, no. 3 (2009): 60-3.

19. "Second National Report on Human Exposure to Environmental Chemicals." Centers for Disease Control and Prevention. 2003.

20. Hauser, Russ, Niels E. Skakkebaek, Ulla Hass, Jorma Toppari, Anders Juul, Anna Maria Andersson, Andreas Kortenkamp, Jerrold J. Heindel, and Leonardo Trasande. "Male Reproductive Disorders, Diseases, and Costs of Exposure to Endocrine-Disrupting Chemicals in the European Union." *The Journal of Clinical Endocrinology & Metabolism* 100, no. 4 (2015): 1267-277.

21. Trasande, Leonardo, R. Thomas Zoeller, Ulla Hass, Andreas Kortenkamp, Philippe Grandjean, John Peterson Myers, Joseph Digangi, Martine Bellanger, Russ Hauser, Juliette Legler, Niels E. Skakkebaek, and Jerrold J. Heindel. "Estimating Burden and Disease Costs of Exposure to Endocrine-Disrupting Chemicals in the European Union." *The Journal of Clinical Endocrinology & Metabolism* 100, no. 4 (2015): 1245-255.

22. Grube, Arthur et al. *Pesticides Industry Sales and Usage 2006 and 2007 Market Estimates.* Washington, D.C., U.S. Environmental Protection Agency, February 2011. http://www.epa.gov/opp00001/pestsales/07pestsales/market_estimates2007.pdf

23. Nussbaum, Robert, Roderick McInnes, and Huntington Willard. *Thompson & Thompson Genetics in Medicine.* Philadelphia: Saunders Elsevier, 2007.

24. Mathur, Sonia. "With Diseases, Genetics Loads The Gun and Environment Pulls the Trigger." The Huffington Post Impact Canada. May 8, 2013. www.huffingtonpost.ca/soania-mathur/avoiding-parkinsons-disease_b_3234752.html.

25. "Neglected Parasitic Infections in the United States." Centers for Disease Control and Prevention.

26. Torrey, E. Fuller, Wendy Simmons, and Robert H. Yolken. "Is Childhood Cat Ownership a Risk Factor for Schizophrenia Later in Life?" *Schizophrenia Research* 165, no. 1 (2015): 1-2.

27. Fasano, Alessio. "Leaky Gut and Autoimmune Diseases." *Clinical Reviews in Allergy & Immunology* 42, no. 1 (2012): 71-8.

28. Kim, Do Young, Junwei Hao, Ruolan Liu, Gregory Turner, Fu-Dong Shi, and Jong M. Rho. "Inflammation-Mediated Memory Dysfunction and Effects of a Ketogenic Diet in a Murine Model of Multiple Sclerosis." *PLoS ONE* 7, no. 5 (2012).

29. Riediger, Natalie D., Rgia A. Othman, Miyoung Suh, and Mohammed H. Moghadasian. "A Systemic Review Of The Roles Of N-3 Fatty Acids In Health And Disease." *Journal of the American Dietetic Association* 109, no. 4 (2009): 668-79.

30. Wahls, Terry L., and Eve Adamson. *The Wahls Protocol: How I Beat Progressive MS Using Paleo Principles and Functional Medicine.* New York: Penguin Group, 2014.

31. Hofmann, Alan F. "Bile Acids: Trying to Understand Their Chemistry and Biology with the Hope of Helping Patients." *Hepatology* 45, no. 9 (2008): 1403-418.

32. Waliszewski, Stefan M., Angel A. Aguirre, Rosa M. Infanzón, and José Siliceo. "Carry-over of Persistent Organochlorine Pesticides through Placenta to Fetus." *Salud Pública Méx Salud Pública De México* 42 (2000): 384-90.

CHAPTER 4

33. Price, Weston, *Nutrition and Physical Degeneration* 6th *Edition.* La Mesa, California: Price-Pottenger Nutrition Foundation, 2000.

34. Schmid, Ron, ND. *The Untold Story of Milk: Green Pastures, Contented Cows and Raw Dairy Products.* White Plains, Maryland: NewTrends Publishing, 2003.

35. "State Studies Milk Problem." *The Lewiston Daily Sun*, February 8, 1945.

36. Fallon, Sally and Mary Enig. *Nourishing Trends: The Cookbook that Challenges Politically Correct Nutrition and the Diet Dictocrats Revised Second Edition.* Washington, D.C.: NewTrends Publishing, 2001.

37. Macdonald, Lauren E., James Brett, David Kelton, Shannon E. Majowicz, Kate Snedeker, and Jan M. Sargeant. "A Systematic Review and Meta-Analysis of the Effects of Pasteurization on Milk Vitamins, and Evidence for Raw Milk Consumption and Other Health-Related Outcomes." *Journal of Food Protection* 74, no. 11 (2011): 1814-832.

38. Sapkota, Amy R., Lisa Y. Lefferts, Shawn McKenzie, and Polly Walker. "What Do We Feed To Food Production Animals? A Review Of Animal Feed Ingredients And Their Potential Impacts On Human Health." *Environmental Health Perspectives* 115, no. 5 (2007): 663-70.

39. Rubin, Jordin. *The Maker's Diet: The 40-Day Health Experience That Will Change Your Life Forever.* Shippenberg, Pennsylvania: Destiny Image Publishiers, Inc., 2005.

40. Hartwig, Dallas, and Melissa Hartwig. *It Starts with Food.* Las Vegas: Victory Belt Publishing, 2012.

41. Buchman, Alan L. "The Addition of Choline to Parenteral Nutrition." *Gastroenterology* 137, no. 5 Suppl. (2009): S119-128.

42. McWilliams, James E. *Just Food: Where Locavores Get It Wrong and How We Can Truly Eat Responsibly.* New York: Little, Brown and Company, 2009.

43. Ostrander, Madeline and Joel Salatin. "Should We Eat Animals?" *Yes! Magazine*, March 2011.

44. Benbrook, Charles et al. *New Evidence Confirms the Nutritional Superiority of Plant-Based Organic Foods.* The Organic Center State of Science Review: Nutritional Superiority of Organic Foods, March 2008. https://www.organic-center.org/reportfiles/5367_Nutrient_Content_SSR_FINAL_V2.pdf.

45. Gupta, Ashish et al. *Impact of Bt Cotton on Farmers' Health (in Barwani and Dhar District of Madhya Pradesh).* Investigation Report, October-December 2005.

46. Kresser, Chris. "RHR: The Truth About Toxic Mercury in Fish." Chris Kresser: Let's Take Back Your Health—Starting Now. October 12, 2012. http://chriskresser.com/the-truth-about-toxic-mercury-in-fish/.

47. Marin, Alinne M. F., Egle M. A. Siqueira, and Sandra F. Arruda. "Minerals, Phytic Acid and Tannin Contents of 18 Fruits from the Brazilian Savanna." *International Journal of Food Sciences and Nutrition* 60, no. 7 Suppl. (2009): 180-90.

48. Davis, William. *Wheat Belly: Lose the Wheat, Lose the Weight, and Find Your Path Back to Health.* Emmaus, Pennsylvania: Rodale, 2011.

49. Punder, Karin De, and Leo Pruimboom. "The Dietary Intake of Wheat and Other Cereal Grains and Their Role in Inflammation." *Nutrients* 5, no. 3 (2013): 771-87.

CHAPTER 5

50. Reynolds, Kelly A., Kristina D. Mena, and Charles P. Gerba. "Risk of Waterborne Illness Via Drinking Water in the United States." *Reviews of Environmental Contamination and Toxicology* 192 (2008): 117-58.

51. Sherman, Paul W., and Jennifer Billing. "Darwinian Gastronomy: Why We Use Spices." *BioScience* 49, no. 6 (1999): 453.

52. *Annual Water Quality Report: Reporting Year 2013*. Gulf Breeze, Florida, Midway Water System, 2014.

53. "A Statement of Concern About Fluoridation." NTEU Chapter 280 – U.S. Environmental Protection Agency. 2003. http://www. nteu280.org/Issues/Fluoride/flouridestatement.htm

54. Yeun, Jane Y., Daniel B. Ornt, Thomas A. Depner, and Maarten W. Taal et al. "Hemodialysis." In *Brenner & Rector's The Kidney*, 2294-2346. Ninth ed. Philadelphia: Saunders Elsevier, 2012.

55. Bond, Tom, Jin Huang, Nigel J.D. Graham, and Michael R. Templeton. "Examining the Interrelationship between DOC, Bromide and Chlorine Dose on DBP Formation in Drinking Water — A Case Study." *Science of The Total Environment* 470-471 (2012): 469-79.

56. Chey, oward, and Susan Buchanan. "Toxins in Everyday Life." *Primary Care: Clinics in Office Practice* 35, no. 4 (2008): 707-27.

57. Roberts, Rebecca. "BPA Exposure and Health Effects: Educating Physicians and Patients." *American Family Physician* 85, no. 11 (2012).

58. Fouque, Denis, William Mitch, and Maarten W. Taal et al. "Diet and Kidney Disease." In *Brenner & Rector's The Kidney*. Ninth ed. Philadelphia: Saunders Elsevier, 2012.

59. Tsindos, Spero. "What Drove Us to Drink 2 Litres of Water a Day?" *Australian and New Zealand Journal of Public Health* 36, no. 3 (2012): 205-07.

60. Valtin, Heinz. ""Drink at Least Eight Glasses of Water a Day." Really? Is There Scientific Evidence for "8 × 8"?" *American Journal of Physiology - Regulatory, Integrative and Comparative Physiology* 283, no. 5 (2002): R993-1004.

61. Meinders, Arend J., and Arend E. Meinders. "How much water do we really need to drink?" *Netherlands Journal of Medicine* 154 (2010): A1757.

CHAPTER 6

62. Teixeira, Pedro J., Eliana V. Carraça, David Markland, Marlene N. Silva, and Richard M. Ryan. "Exercise, Physical Activity, and Self-determination Theory: A Systematic Review." *International Journal of Behavioral Nutrition and Physical Activity* 9 (2012):78.

63. Moore, Steven C. et al. "Leisure Time Physical Activity of Moderate to Vigorous Intensity and Mortality: A Large Pooled Cohort Analysis." *PLoS Medicine* (November 2012): E1001335.

64. Cooper, Dan M. et al. "Dangerous Exercise: Lessons Learned From Dysregulated Inflammatory Responses To Physical Activity." *Journal of Applied Physiology* 103, no. 2 (2007): 700-09.

65. Lyod Jr., Allen V. "Adrenal Fatigue." *International Journal of Pharmaceutical Compounding* 17, no. 1 (2013): 39-44.

66. Schneider, Tom. *A Physician's Apology: Are WE Making You Sick?* Pensacola, Florida: Indigo River Publishing 2013.

67. Lane, Amy R., Joseph W. Duke, and Anthony C. Hackney. "Influence of Dietary Carbohydrate Intake on the Free Testosterone: Cortisol Ratio Responses to Short-term Intensive Exercise Training." *European Journal of Applied Physiology* 108, no. 6 (2010): 1125-131.

68. Takase, Kanae. "Prospective Study of the Relation Between Exercise Performance for Health Promotion, Self-Efficacy, and Outcome Expectation of Elderly People." *Japanese Journal of Geriatrics* 44, no. 1 (2007): 107-16.

69. Do, Barbara T., Jennifer M. Hootman, Charles G. Helmick, and Teresa J. Brady. "Monitoring Healthy People 2010 Arthritis Management Objectives: Education and Clinician Counseling for Weight Loss and Exercise." *The Annals of Family Medicine* 9, no. 2 (2011): 136-41.

70. Rose, Debra J., and Danielle Hernandez. "The Role of Exercise in Fall Prevention for Older Adults." *Clinics in Geriatric Medicine* 26, no. 4 (2010): 607-31.

71. Horne, Jim. "Exercise Benefits for the Aging Brain Depend on the Accompanying Cognitive Load: Insights from Sleep Electroencephalogram." *Sleep Medicine* 14, no. 11 (2013): 1208-213.

72. Sivasankaran, Satish, Suzanne Pollard-Quintner, Rajesh Sachdeva, Jaime Pugeda, Sheik M. Hoq, and Stuart W. Zarich. "The Effect of a Six-Week Program of Yoga and Meditation on Brachial Artery Reactivity: Do Psychosocial Interventions Affect Vascular Tone?" *Clinical Cardiology* 29, no. 9 (2006): 393-98.

73. Kerr, John H., and George Kuk. "The Effects of Low and High Intensity Exercise on Emotions, Stress and Effort." *Psychology of Sport and Exercise* 2, no. 3 (2001): 173-86.

74. Nidhi, Ram, Venkatram Padmalatha, Raghuram Nagarathna, and Amritanshu Ram. "Effect of a Yoga Program on Glucose Metabolism and Blood Lipid Levels in Adolescent Girls with Polycystic Ovary Syndrome." *International Journal of Gynecology & Obstetrics* 118, no. 1 (2012): 37-41.

75. Boon, Brooke. *Holy Yoga: Exercise for the Christian Body and Soul.* New York: FaithWords, 2007.

76. Freedman, Francoise B. *Yoga & Pilates for Everyone.* London: Hermes House, 2005.

77. Louveau, Antoine et al. "Structural and functional features of central nervous system lymphatic vessels." *Nature* (June 2015): 337-41.

CHAPTER 7

78. Ishikawa, Hayato, David A. Colby, Shigeki Seto, Porino Va, Annie Tam, Hiroyuki Kakei, Thomas J. Rayl, Inkyu Hwang, and Dale L. Boger. "Total Synthesis of Vinblastine, Vincristine, Related Natural Products, and Key Structural Analogues." *Journal of the American Chemical Society* 131, no. 13 (2009): 4904-916.

79. Rajabalian, Saeed. "Methanolic extract of Teucrium polium L. potentiates the cytotoxic and apoptotic effects of anticancer drugs of vincristine, vinblastine and doxorubicin against a panel

of cancerous cell lines." *Experimental Oncology* 30, no. 2 (2008): 133-8.

80. Hobbs, Christopher. *Herbal Remedies for Dummies*. Foster City, California: IDG Books Worldwide, 1998.

81. Shiina, Yumi et al. "Relaxation Effects of Lavender Aromatherapy Improve Coronary Flow Velocity Reserve in Healthy Men Evaluated by Transthoracic Doppler Echocardiography." *International Journal of Cardiology* 129, no. 2 (2008): 193-97.

82. Karpanen, Tarja et al. "Antimicrobial Efficacy of Chlorhexidine Digluconate Alone and In Combination with Eucalyptus Oil, Tea Tree Oil and Thymol Against Planktonic and Biofilm Cultures of Staphylococcus Epidermidis. *Journal of Antimicrobal Chemotherapy* 62, no. 5 (2008): 1031-36.

83. Steflitsch, Michaela and Wolfgang Steflitsch. "Clinical Aromatherapy." *Journal of Men's Health* 5, no. 1 (2008): 74-85.

84. Coulter, Harris. *Divided Legacy, Volume II: A History of the Schism in Medical Thought*. Washington D.C.: North Atlantic Books, 2000.

85. Hahnemann, Samuel. *Organon of Medicine*. Los Angeles: J.P. Tarcher, 1982.

86. Bonamin, Leoni V. et al. "Very High Dilutions of Dexamethasone Inhibit Its Pharmacological Effects in Vivo." *British Homoeopathic Journal* 90 (2001): 198-203.

87. Gladstar, Rosemary. *Rosemary Gladstar's Medicinal Herbs: A Beginner's Guide*. North Adams, Massachusetts: Storey Publishing, 2012.

88. Mills, Simon and Kerry Bone. *The Essential Guide to Herbal Safety*. St. Louis: Elsevier, Inc., 2005.

89. Vervelle, A. et al. "Mouthwash Solutions with Microencapsuled Natural Extracts: Efficiency for Dental Plaque and Gingivitis." *Revue de Stomatologie et de Chirurgie Maxillo-Faciale* 111, no. 3 (2010): 148-51.

90. Mandel, Abigail L., and Paul A. S. Breslin. "High Endogenous Salivary Amylase Activity Is Associated with Improved Glycemic Homeostasis following Starch Ingestion in Adults." *Journal of Nutrition* 142, no. 5 (2012): 853-58.

91. Haydel, Shelley E., Christine Remenih, and Lynda B. Williams. "Broad-spectrum in Vitro Antibacterial Activities of Clay Minerals against Antibiotic-susceptible and Antibiotic-resistant Bacterial Pathogens." *Journal of Antimicrobial Chemotherapy* 61, no. 2 (2008): 353-61.

92. Lapus, Robert Michael. "Activated Charcoal for Pediatric Poisonings: The Universal Antidote?" *Current Opinion in Pediatrics* 19, no. 2 (2007): 216-22.

93. Essen, Marina Rode Von, Martin Kongsbak, Peter Schjerling, Klaus Olgaard, Niels Ødum, and Carsten Geisler. "Vitamin D Controls T Cell Antigen Receptor Signaling and Activation of Human T Cells." *Nature Immunology* (2010), 344-49.

94. Chemych, Mykola et al. "Morphological Changes of the Intestine in Experimental Acute Intestinal Infection in the Treatment of Colloidal Silver." *Georgian Med News* 207 (2010): 63-7.

95. Cha, Kwang Y., Daniel P. Wirth, Rogerio A. Lobo. "Does Prayer Influence the Success of In Vitro Fertilization–Embryo Transfer? Report of a Masked, Randomized Trial." *The Journal of Reproductive Medicine* 46 (2001): 781-787.

CHAPTER 8

96. Lloyd, Bradley D. et al. "Recurrent and Injurious Falls in the Year Following Hip Fracture: A Prospective Study of Incidence and Risk Factors From the Sarcopenia and Hip Fracture Study." *The Journals of Gerontology Series A: Biological Sciences and Medical Sciences* 64, no. 5 (2009): 599-609.

97. Vestergaard, Peter et al. "Proton Pump Inhibitors, Histamine H2 Receptor Antagonists, and Other Antacid Medications and the Risk of Fracture." *Calcified Tissue International* 79, no. 2 (2006): 76-83.

98. Vargas, Ivan, and Nestor Lopez-Duran. "Dissecting the Impact of Sleep and Stress on the Cortisol Awakening Response in Young Adults." *Psychoneuroendocrinology* 40 (2014): 10-16.

99. Roehrs, Timothy, and T. Roth. "Caffeine: Sleep And Daytime Sleepiness." *Sleep Medicine Reviews* 12, no. 2 (2008): 153-62.

100. Kimberly, Burkhart, and Phelps James R. "Amber Lenses To Block Blue Light And Improve Sleep: A Randomized Trial." *Chronobiology International* 26, no. 8 (2009): 1602-612.

101. Teekachunhatean, Supanimit et al. "Antioxidant Effects after Coffee Enema or Oral Coffee Consumption in Healthy Thai Male Volunteers." *Human & Experimental Toxicology* 31, no. 7 (2012): 643-51.

102. Cassileth, Barrie. "Gerson Regimen." *Oncology* 24, no. 2 (2010): 201.

103. Alcantara, Joel, and James Davis. "The Chiropractic Care Of Children With Attention-Deficit/Hyperactivity Disorder: A Retrospective Case Series." *EXPLORE: The Journal of Science and Healing* 6, no. 3 (2010): 173-82.

104. Lis-Balchin, Maria, and Stephen Hart. "A Preliminary Study of the Effect of Essential Oils on Skeletal and Smooth Muscle in Vitro." *Journal of Ethnopharmacology* 58, no. 3 (1997): 183-87.

105. Walker, Bruce F., Simon D. French, William Grant, and Sally Green. "Combined Chiropractic Interventions for Low-Back Pain." *Cochrane Database of Systematic Reviews* 4 (2010).

106. Grieves, Brian, J. Michael Menke, and Kevin J. Pursel. "Cost Minimization Analysis of Low Back Pain Claims Data for Chiropractic Vs Medicine in a Managed Care Organization." *Journal of Manipulative and Physiological Therapeutics* 32, no. 9 (2009): 734-39.

107. Skargren, Elisabeth I., Per G. Carlsson, and Birgitta E. Öberg. "One-Year Follow-up Comparison of the Cost and Effectiveness of Chiropractic and Physiotherapy as Primary Management for Back Pain." *Spine* 23, no. 17 (1998): 1875-883.

108. "Autoimmune Disease in Women." AARDA. August 29, 2013. http://www.aarda.org/autoimmune-information/autoimmune-disease-in-women/.

109. Nambudripad, Devi S. *NAET: Say Goodbye to Asthma: A Revolutionary Treatment for Allergy-Based Asthma and Other Respiratory Disorders*. McHenry, Illinois: Delta Publishing Company, 2003.

110. Weintraub, M., and Marc Micozzi. "Biophysical Devices: Electricity, Light, and Magnetism." In *Fundamentals of Complementary and Alternative Medicine*. 4th ed. St. Louis: Saunders, 2011.

111. Amri, H., and Marc Micozzi. "*Neurohumoral Physiology and Psychoneuroimmunology*." In *Fundamentals of Complementary and Alternative Medicine*. 4th ed. St. Louis: Saunders, 2011.

112. Rindfleisch, J. Adam. "Biofield Therapies: Energy Medicine and Primary Care." *Primary Care: Clinics in Office Practice* 37, no. 1 (2010): 165-79.

113. Hughes, Mark. "Olfaction, Emotion & the Amygdala: Arousal-Dependent Modulation of Long-Term Autobiographical Memory and its Association with Olfaction: Beginning to Unravel the Proust Phenomenon?" *Impulse* 1, no. 1 (2013): 1-58.

114. Barbasio, Chiara, and Antonella Granieri. "Emotion Regulation and Mental Representation of Attachment in Patients With Systemic Lupus Erythematosus." *The Journal of Nervous and Mental Disease* 201, no. 4 (2014): 304-10.

115. Kaliman, Perla, María Jesús Álvarez-López, Marta Cosín-Tomás, Melissa A. Rosenkranz, Antoine Lutz, and Richard J. Davidson. "Rapid Changes in Histone Deacetylases and Inflammatory Gene Expression in Expert Meditators." *Psychoneuroendocrinology* 40 (2014): 96-107.

116. Crum, Alia J., William R. Corbin, Kelly D. Brownell, and Peter Salovey. "Mind over Milkshakes: Mindsets, Not Just Nutrients, Determine Ghrelin Response." *Health Psychology* 30, no. 4 (2011): 424-29.

117. Chang, Bei-Hung, Debra Jones, Ann Hendricks, Ulrike Boehmer, Joseph S. Locastro, and Mara Slawsky. "Relaxation Response for Veterans Affairs Patients With Congestive Heart Failure: Results From a Qualitative Study Within a Clinical Trial." *Preventive Cardiology* 7, no. 2 (2004): 64-70.

APPENDIX

118. Liener, Irvin. "Implications of Antinutritional Components in Soybean Foods." *Critical Reviews in Food Science Nutrition* 34, no. 1 (1994): 31-67.

119. Shike, Moshe, et al. "The Effects of Soy Supplementation on Gene Expression in Breast Cancer: A Randomized Placebo-Controlled Study." *Journal of the National Cancer Institute* 106, no. 9 (2014).

120. Sathyapalan, Thozhukat, et al. "The Effect of Soy Phytoestrogen Supplementation on Thyroid Status and Cardiovascular Risk Markers in Patients with Subclinical Hypothyroidism: A Randomized, Double-Blind, Crossover Study." *The Journal of Clinical Endocrinology and Metabolism* 96, no 5 (2011): 1442-9.

121. Conrad, Susan, et al. "Soy Formula Complicates Management of Congenital Hypothyroidism." *Archives of Disease in Childhood* 89, no 1 (2004):37-40.

Resources

Blogs

- The Grecian Garden thegreciangarden.com You're welcome to join a closed Facebook group where I post exclusive content for those who purchased my book: on.fb.me/1ZMuiVS
- GFE glutenfreeeasily.com
- Rubies and Radishes rubiesandradishes.com
- Paleo OMG paleoomg.com
- Elana's Pantry elanaspantry.com
- Kitchen Stewardship kitchenstewardship.com
- Natural Fertility naturalfertilityandwellness.com
- Ancestral Health ancestralizeme.com
- Diane Sanfilippo balancedbites.com
- Junior Desouza juniordesouza.com
- Grass-fed Girl grassfedgirl.com
- The Nourishing Home thenourishinghome.com
- Paleo Eats paleoeats.com
- Delicious Obsessions deliciousobsessions.com
- Melanie's communications melaniespeaking.com

Body Products

- Primal Life Organics' primallifeorganics.com All natural skin care products.
- Red Apple redapplelipstick.com Non-toxic makeup

- 100% Pure* 100percentpure.com Non-toxic makeup
- Jurlique* jurlique.com Non-toxic skin care products
- Jane Iredale janeiredale.com Non-toxic makeup
- Primal Pit Paste™ primalpitpaste.com Natural deodorant
- Aubrey Organics* aubrey-organics.com All natural skin care products.
- Peacekeeper Causmetics* iamapeacekeeper.com All natural make-up
- Tarte tartecosmetics.com All natural make-up
- Living Libations livinglibations.com Holistic dental care
- Ener-G-Polari-T™ energpolarit.com EMF protection

Find a Practitioner

- Bioset bioset.net
- Nutrition Response Testing℠ unsinc.info
- Walsh Institute walshinstitute.org
- Kalish Method kalishinstitute.com
- Functional RD integrativerd.org

Food

- Tin Star Foods tinstarfoods.com
- OMghee omghee.com
- Love Bean Fudge* lovebeanfudge.com
- U.S. Wellness Meats™ grasslandbeef.com
- Kasandrinos Olive Oil kasandrinos.com
- Eat Wild* eatwild.com
- Primal Kitchen Mayo™ primalkitchen.com
- Local Harvest localharvest.org

Functional Movement

- MovNat* movnat.com
- T-Tapp™ t-tapp.com
- Revelation Wellness revelationwellness.org
- Holy Yoga™ holyyoga.net

Home Products

- Natural House naturalhouse.com Probiotic and non toxic house cleaners
- Naturalizing Water System waterforwellness.us Water filters
- New Wave Enviro newwaveenviro.com Shower filters
- Berkey˙ berkeywater.com Water filters
- Ener-G-Polari-T™ energpolarit.com EMF Protection
- Vita Clay˙ vitaclaychef.com Lead free clay pot crock pot
- Pickl-it˙ pickl-it.com Cultured vegetable tools

Natural Health Websites

- Weston A Price Foundation˙ westonaprice.org
- Paleo FX paleofx.com
- American Council of Holistic Medicine theachm.org
- American College of Healthcare Sciences achs.edu
- MTHFR.net
- Chris Kresser chriskesser.com
- Dr. Justin Marchegiani justinhealth.com
- Lynne Farrow lynnefarrow.net Iodine supplementation
- Mark's Daily Apple marksdailyapple.com
- Underground Wellness undergroundwellness.com
- Dave Asprey bulletproofexec.com
- Daniel Vitalis danielvitalis.com

Nutrition Programs

- Whole 30˙ whole30.com
- The 21 Day Sugar Detox™ 21daysugardetox.com
- AIP thepaleomom.com Dr. Sarah Ballantyne
- Body Ecology bodyecology.com
- Gut and Psychology Syndrome gapsdiet.com
- Specific Carbohydrate Diet™ breakingtheviciouscycle.info

Supplement Companies

- Designs for Health* designsforhealth.com
- Seeking Health* seekinghealth.com
- Garden of Life* gardenoflife.com
- Green Pastures™ greenpasture.org
- Prescript Assist™ prescript-assist.com
- Mountain Rose™ herbs
- Rocky Mountain Oils rockymountainoils.com
- Vibrant Blue Oils vibrantblueoils
- Perfect Dessicated Liver perfectsupplements.com
- Vital Nutrients vitalnutrients.net
- Klaire Labs* klaire.com
- The Synergy Company™ thesynergycompany.com
- Douglas Labs* douglaslabs.com

Glossary

active placebo affect	Often associated with the side effects of psychiatric drugs: a new substance causes noticeable change. This convinces the test subject that they are receiving something to help with symptoms and results in a positive effect for researchers in a double blind study. Source: http://stlr.org/2010/12/04/the-active-placebo-effect-patent-eligible-subject-matter/
acupuncture	A technique in which practitioners stimulate specific points on the body—most often by inserting thin needles through the skin. It is one of the practices used in *traditional Chinese medicine*...to help ease types of pain that are often chronic such as low-back pain, neck pain, and osteoarthritis/knee pain. It also may help reduce the frequency of tension headaches and prevent migraine headaches. Source National Institutes of Health (NIH).
alternative medicine	Healing systems not included in conventional, allopathic medical training, although they may complement it.

arachidonic acid	Otherwise known as Omega-6 fatty acid. Found primarily in fatty red meats, egg yolks and organ meats, this particular polyunsaturated fat may be the most dangerous fat as too much arachidonic acid can lead to health risks including cardiovascular issues. Sources include PubChem.
autoimmune diseases	An autoimmune disorder occurs when the body's immune system attacks and destroys healthy body tissue by mistake. There are more than 80 types of autoimmune disorders, e.g., type I diabetes, rheumatoid arthritis, lupus, and multiple sclerosis. Source: NIH
Ayurvedic medicine	Originated in India more than 3000 years ago, it remains one of the country's traditional health care systems. Its concepts about health and disease promote the use of herbal compounds, special diets, and other unique health practices. Source: NIH
biohack	Use a combination of medical, nutritional and electronic techniques to manage health.
Blastocystis hominis	A microscopic parasite that may cause diarrhea, abdominal pain or other gastrointestinal problems. Source Mayo Clinic
Body Ecology diet	A back-to-basics natural approach to cleanse, restore, and maintain the important "inner ecology" of your body. The diet is based on the addition of cultured foods, the use of "good" fats and the dramatic reduction of carbohydrates and sugar. Source: Bodyecology.com
BPA	Bisphenol A found in polycarbonate plastics used in food and beverage containers. Exposure to BPA is a concern because of possible health effects of BPA on the endocrine system, the brain, behavior and prostate gland of fetuses, infants and children. Source: Mayo Clinic.

bradykinins	Formed locally in injured tissue, acts in vasodilation of small arterioles and is considered to play a part in the inflammatory process. Source: Merriam-Webster.
Candida	Candida is a genus of yeasts. Normally it is a necessary part of the normal flora of the gut that aids in digestion. When uncontrolled or overgrown, it is the most common cause of fungal infections worldwide. Sources include: Wikipedia.
case study	A research method often used in alternative medicine: accounts for all the variables in an individual situation. Not always applicable to a population as it may be for the outliers of a more general study.
chronic Lyme	The belief that the spirochetes from ticks causing Lyme disease resist conventional treatment options and result in deteriorating health.
cortisol	Called the stress hormone, elevated levels interfere with learning and memory, lower immune function and bone density, increase weight gain, blood pressure, cholesterol, heart disease, and much more. Exercise does a great job reducing and normalizing cortisol levels. This makes it easier to lose weight, improve your sleep, makes you feel more relaxed and able to handle all of life's changes. Source: psychologytoday.com.
COX inhibitors	COX-2 selective *inhibitors* are a form of non-steroidal anti-inflammatory drug (NSAID) that directly targets COX-2, an enzyme responsible for inflammation and pain. Source: http://my.clevelandclinic.org/health/ drugs_devices_supplements/hic_COX-2_ Nonsteroidal_Anti-inflammatory_Drugs_NSAIDs

craniosacral manipulation	Originates from the osteopathic philosophy and is a gentle, hands on approach to release tensions in the soft tissues that surround the central nervous system.
crossfit	Combines strength training, explosive plyometrics, speed training, Olympic- and power-style weight lifting, kettle bells, body weight exercises, gymnastics, and endurance exercise and targets the major components of physical fitness. Source: WebMD
detox	Tissue and organs constantly transform harmful chemicals into inactive metabolites. A new diet or supplement can assist, but cleansing is rarely a long-term solution.
DHEA	A natural steroid and precursor hormone produced by the adrenal glands located on top of the kidneys. Long term use as a supplement may cause certain cancers, heart disease and stroke.
diffusing	Dispersing essential oils so their aroma fills an area, often via humidified air.
double-blinded research	A scientific standard: refers to studies where neither study designers nor cohorts know when the studied variable is in play.
earthing	Going barefoot outside allows your body to naturally receive and become charged with an unlimited supply of free electrons that will correct any electron deficiencies and free radical excesses, restoring a natural electrical state. Earthing has been found to promote intriguing physiological changes, resulting, among other things, in better sleep and reduced pain. Sources include http://www.ncbi.nlm.nih.gov/pmc

Eastern medicine	A holistic philosophy based on the healing practices of traditional cultures rather than the scientific method and standard American/European care.
EMF	Electromagnetic fields (EMFs) are areas of energy that surround all electrical devices and sources of electricity.
emotional release work	Techniques to release emotions buried within the body that cause changes in internal chemical reactions. These can lead to serious illness, including cancer, arthritis, and many types of chronic illnesses. Sources include mkprojects.com.
energy medicine	Modalities such as Reiki and Therapeutic Touch designed to improve health apart from manual therapies or other alternative techniques.
Environmental Working Group (EWG)	An American environmental organization that specializes in research and advocacy in the areas of toxic chemicals, agricultural subsidies, public lands, and corporate accountability. Source: ewg.org.
Epstein Barre virus	Epstein-Barr virus (EBV), also known as human herpesvirus 4, is a member of the herpes virus family. It is one of the most common human viruses and can cause infectious mononucleosis, also called mono, and other illnesses. Source: Centers for Disease Control.
essential oils	A concentrated liquid containing volatile aroma compounds from plants. Essential oils are primarily used to promote healing, reducing toxin loads, and cleaning. Sources include floracopeia.com.
functional medicine	Similar to the fusion of Western and Eastern thought known as integrative medicine. Focuses on genetics, optimal laboratory values, and practical, individualized care.

GAPS diet	A diet designed to heal a leaky gut reduce toxins, and eliminate allergens. Removes the user from the typical modern diet full of sugar, artificial and processed ingredients, and other harmful foods. Source: gapsdiet.com
ghrelin	Called the hunger hormone, it helps to regulate hunger and is involved in the complex system of energy homeostasis. Numerous technical sources.
glycerite	A traditional *glycerite* is a fluid extract of an herb or other medicinal substance made using glycerin instead of alcohol as the majority of the fluid extraction medium.
GMOs	Genetically modified organisms, plants or animals. Most are designed to improve yields and reduce susceptibility to disease. Numerous sources.
hair mineral analysis testing	Standard for biological monitoring of trace elements and toxic substances.
heavy metals	Refers to unhealthy levels of mercury, lead, or aluminum that remain in the body through fillings or environmental exposure. Depending on the practitioner, the best discovery method is Doctor's Data Urine Test or hair testing.
holistic nutrition	The modern natural approach to developing a healthy balanced diet while taking into account the person as whole. Source nanp.org (National Association of Nutrition Professionals)
homeopathic	Homeopathy is a safe, gentle, and natural system of healing that works with your body to relieve symptoms, restore itself, and improve your overall health through the use of homeopathics (low dose remedies). Sources include livestrong.com.
homocysteine levels	High levels of homocysteine are related to the early development of heart and blood vessel disease. Source WebMD

IBS	Irritable bowel syndrome (IBS) is a common disorder that affects the large intestine (colon). Irritable bowel syndrome commonly causes cramping, abdominal pain, bloating, gas, diarrhea and constipation. IBS is a chronic condition that you will need to manage long term. Source: Mayo Clinic.
inflammation	The body's attempt at self-protection when something harmful or irritating affects a part of our body. Sometimes inflammation is self-perpetuating and can cause further issues, including some as major as cancers, rheumatoid arthritis, atherosclerosis, periodontitis, and hay fever. Source: Medical News Today.
kinesiology	Also known as human kinetics, it is the scientific study of human movement.
Leaky Gut Syndrome	A predisposition for food sensitivities, malnutrition, infections and auto-immune inflammation, and malnutrition caused by a permeable gut lining. Sources include mdheal.com
l-glutamine	Glutamine is the most abundant amino acid (building block of protein) in the body. It is important for removing excess ammonia (a common waste product in the body). It also helps your immune system function and appears to be needed for normal brain function and digestion. L-glutamine can be used as a supplement if levels of glutamine drop after major injuries, surgery, infections, and prolonged stress. Source: University of Maryland Medical Center.
leptin	Called the satiety hormone, it helps to regulate fat storage and energy expenditures.

liver metabolism	Has two phases and varies among individuals, especially in those on multiple medications and with chronic diseases. This is why individual genetic and diagnostic testing is superior to standardized methods. Biliary, lung, blood, and kidney metabolism all use different methods to detoxify and excrete substances.
magnesium RBC	Blood test to determine magnesium levels. Magnesium is an essential trace element. Deficiency leads to irritability, neuromuscular abnormalities, cardiac and renal damage. Its salts are used as antacids and cathartics. Excessive amount may cause CNS depression, loss of muscle tone, respiratory and cardiac arrest. Source questdiagnostics.com.
meridians	Originating in Chinese medicine, meridians are the pathways of qi (chi) and blood flow through the body. Any break in the flow is an indication of imbalance. Healing is based on the concept that an insufficient supply of qi makes a person vulnerable to disease. Sources include healingabout.com
meta-analysis	A method for systematically combining pertinent qualitative and quantitative study data from several selected studies to develop a single conclusion that has greater statistical power. Sources include: *himmelfarb.gwu.edu*
methylation defects	Methylation occurs when the body takes one substance and turns it into another, so it is detoxified and can be excreted from the body. Faulty methylation has been linked to heart disease, stroke, neural tube defects, and Alzheimer's disease. Numerous sources.
millet	A grain rich in B vitamins (especially niacin, B6 and folic acid), calcium, iron, potassium, magnesium, and zinc.

MTHFR	A gene that when defective or mutated can result in numerous diseases as diverse as Parkinson's, autism, and certain cancers. Sources include: mthfr.net.
muscle testing	Non-invasive evaluation of the body's needs to pinpoint foods and supplements that can restore balance.
natural health	Focusing on everyday living and the use of accessible, gentle, gradual, and balanced modalities to achieve wellness without the risk of toxic effects.
Omega-3 fatty acids	Found in fish and plant sources such as nuts and seeds, most people don't have enough of this. Sources include: WebMD
Omega-6 fatty acids	Another essential fatty acid. Omega 3 and Omega 6 Fatty Acids help lower the risk of heart disease. Some studies suggest these fats may also protect against type 2 diabetes, Alzheimer's disease, and age-related brain decline. Sources include: WebMD
osteopathy	A type of complementary and alternative medicine which primarily consists of moving, stretching and massaging a person's muscles and joints.
oxidative stress	A disturbance in the balance between the production of reactive oxygen species (free radicals) and antioxidant defenses. Some studies indicate, among other things, it may have a role in the production of tissue damage in diabetes mellitus. Source: http://www.ncbi.nlm.nih.gov/pubmed/10693912.
Paleo Auto Immune Protocol	Besides avoiding grains, legumes, dairy, refined sugars, modern vegetable oils, and processed food chemicals, this diet also avoids eggs, nuts, seeds, nightshades, non-nutritive sweeteners, and other potential irritants. Source: Sarah Ballantyne, PhD

Paleo Diet	Paleo is based upon the fundamental concept that the optimal diet is the one to which we are genetically adapted. Organ meats, healthy saturated fats, and organic fruits and vegetables are preferred. The therapeutic effect is supported by randomized controlled human trials. Source: Loren Cordain, PhD
parabens	Preservatives used in cosmetics and some pharmaceuticals to prevent growth of microbes.
parasitic infection	Parasites are microorganisms that live off of other organisms, or hosts, to survive. Some parasites don't affect the host. Others grow, reproduce, or give off toxins that make the host sick resulting in a parasitic infection. Source: healthline.com
prostaglandins	Lipids released as a result of irritation or injury, they play a key role in the inflammatory response and have been implicated in the pathogeneses of arthritis, cancer and stroke, as well as in neurodegenerative and cardiovascular disease. Source: NIH
quercetin	Quercetin is a plant pigment (flavonoid). Found in many plants and foods, such as red wine, onions, green tea, apples, and berries, it has antioxidant and anti-inflammatory effects and is used for many medical conditions. Source: Mills, Simon & Bone, Kerry. (2010). The Essential Guide to Herbal Safety. Elsevier: Philadelphia.
quinoa	High in protein and fiber, quinoa is a grain crop grown primarily for its edible seeds and high nutritional value.
reflexology	Acupressure on the feet.
saliva hormone testing	Often involves spitting into specimen bottles at prescribed intervals to determine fluctuating hormone levels; does not measure total amounts of hormones.

SCD protocol	Designed to help people with bowel disorders, the Specific Carbohydrate Diet limits the use of complex carbohydrates (disaccharides and polysaccharides). Monosaccharides are allowed, and various foods including fish, aged cheese and honey are included. Prohibited foods include cereal grains, potatoes and lactose-containing dairy products. Source: Breakingtheviciouscycle.info
snake oil	Unproven or overused cure-all with potential harmful effects.
SNP	Single Nucleotide Polymorphism is a variation in the DNA sequence discoverable by genetic testing. Mapping out a person's genome is most useful in a holistic context of their environment, diet, etc.
stool testing	Identifies intestinal infections and their source (bacteria, parasites, etc.).
tapping	A natural technique to help relax and clear undesired emotions by tapping (with your finger) along the meridian lines or acupuncture points. Source: Feinstein, David (December 2012). "Acupoint stimulation in treating psychological disorders: Evidence of efficacy". *Review of General Psychology* 16 (4): 364–380. doi:10.1037/a0028602
toxic burden	Toxic chemicals, both naturally occurring and man-made, are inhaled, swallowed in contaminated food and water, or in some cases, absorbed through skin. Continuous exposure to such chemicals can create a "persistent" body (or toxic burden) that can cause a long list of health problems. Sources include: NIH

T-Tapp exercise	A rehabilitative physical therapy approach to fitness that delivers muscle density rather than bulk and focuses on inches lost instead of weight lost. Exercises all parts of the muscle (origin, insertion, and belly). Source: t-tapp.com
wellness	A progressive, all-encompassing state of health for mind, soul, and body.
Weston A Price Foundation	An organization dedicated to "restoring nutrient-dense foods to the American diet through education, research and activism."